Renal Anemia

Conflicts and Controversies

Renal Anemia
Conflicts and Controversies

Edited by

Onyekachi Ifudu

Associate Professor of Medicine
Director, Inpatient Dialysis Services
SUNY Downstate Medical Center, Brooklyn, New York

KAP ARCHIEF

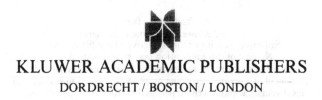

KLUWER ACADEMIC PUBLISHERS
DORDRECHT / BOSTON / LONDON

Library of Congress Cataloging-in-Publication Data is available.

ISBN 978-90-481-6045-7

Published by Kluwer Academic Publishers,
PO Box 17, 3300 AA Dordrecht, The Netherlands.

Sold and distributed in North, Central and South America
by Kluwer Academic Publishers
101 Philip Drive, Norwell, MA 02018, USA

In all other countries, sold and distributed
by Kluwer Academic Publishers, Distribution Center,
PO Box 322, 3300 AH Dordrecht, The Netherlands

Printed on acid-free paper

Dedication

To Munachiso "my moon", and Audrey for bringing such joy.

Table of Contents

Introduction to the Conference

Eli A. Friedman

Nephrology evolved as a discipline of value to sick people as the consequence of sometimes startling unexpected vanguard advances that transformed the kidney doctor from a sideline observer to an active interventionist. As a prime example of the transformation in practice that might derive from a single experiment reflect on Willem J. Kolff's 1943 invention of a practical artificial kidney using sausage casing and cellophane. At once, uremia was in acute renal failure was converted from a frustratingly inexorable march culminating in death to a signal for repetitive treatment.

Similarly, less than a generation later, Belding H. Scribner devised a regimen for repetitive access to arterial and venous blood thereby permitting maintenance hemodialysis, a therapy that sustains more than half-a-million individuals who would otherwise have died from so called end-stage renal disease (ESRD). Contemporaneous with construction of hemodialysis protocols for ESRD, successful kidney transplantation and peritoneal dialysis were introduced affording a menu of choices for formerly hopeless ESRD patients.

Once life despite ESRD was proven extendable – a miraculous accomplishment vividly recalled by those old enough to have experienced the therapeutic triumph impact on their patients – attention shifted to the quality and complexity of dialysis-salvaged lives. Recognition of the adverse impact of hypertension within the first years of applying maintenance hemodialysis was followed by appreciation of the danger imposed by hyperphosphatemia and aluminum contaminated dialysate.(and later phosphate binders). By the end of a decade of maintenance hemodialysis, antihypertensive medications along with unpalatable phosphate binders became bedrock accompaniments of dialysis treatment. Two pervasive problems limited rehabilitation in maintenance hemodialysis as the 1980s began: delivery of insufficient dialysis and anemia.

Clear correlation between the length of dialysis treatments and survival as well as comparisons between "good" and "bad" dialysis facilities led to standards in the form of "quality assurance" with a targeted minimum of four hours of hemodialysis per treatment. Improvement in anemia eluded nephrologists who tried and discontinued periodic transfusions of eyrthocytes, androgens and cobalt. And then, the astonishing and profound effect of injected erythropoietin eliminated severe anemia in the absence of infections, active bleeding, extrarenal diseases, and primary hematologic disorders. By the end of the 20th Century, erythropoietin was a fixed element of dialytic therapy for about 90% of American dialysis patients at an annual cost in excess of $3 billion.

Still, something was not right about our use of erythropoietin. Dose response curves were highly variable and the perceived need for and response to supplemental iron was inconstant and unpredictable. Two competing explanations were considered: 1) Many dialysis patients are iron deficient though treated with oral iron supplements, affording strong evidence for the hypothesis that dialysis patients must receive iron parenterally changing usual practice. 2) Insufficient dialysis blunts erythropoietin efficacy and may be masked by some response in terms of hemoglobin/hematocrit rise when iron is administered. These Conference Proceedings address implementation of the wondrous benefits that can be bestowed by erythropoietin usage. Considering the expense and inconvenience imposed on patients by an established program of erythropoietin treatment, it is appropriate that all those who prescribe the hormone optimize its application and benefits. The pages that follow represent the efforts of accomplished workers who strive to attain this objective.

Conference Participants: Brooklyn, New York, USA, September 21, 2001

Program Director
Onyekachi Ifudu, M.D., M.Sc
Associate Professor of Medicine
Director, Inpatient Dialysis Services
SUNY Downstate Medical Center
Brooklyn, New York

Guest Faculty

Adeera Levin, M.D.
Associate Professor of Medicine
Program Director, Nephrology
St. Paul's Hospital, Vancouver, Canada
President, Canadian Society of
   Nephrology

Chaim Charytan, M.D.
Chief, Renal Division
NY Hospital Medical Center of Queens
Clinical Professor of Medicine
Cornell University College of Medicine

Steven Fishbane, M.D.
Associate Professor of Medicine
SUNY Stony Brook
Associate Chief of Nephrology
Winthrop-University Hospital, Mineola

Jill Lindberg, M.D.
Director of Nephrology Research
Director of Metabolic and Bone Clinics
Associate Section Head – Hemodialysis
Ochsner Foundation Hospital,
   New Orleans

Iain C. Macdougall, BSc, M.D., F.R.C.P.
Consultant Nephrologist
King's College Hospital, London

**Wendy L. St. Peter, Pharm.D, F.C.C.P,
B.C.P.S.**
Associate Professor
College of Pharmacy, University of
   Minnesota
Co-investigator, Nephrology Analytical
   Services
Hennepin County Medical Center,
   Minneapolis

Rebecca J. Schmidt, D.O., F.A.C.P.
Associate Professor of Medicine
West Virginia University School of Medi-
   cine

SUNY Downstate Medical Center Faculty

Clinton Brown, M.D.
Assistant Professor of Medicine
Director, Ambulatory Dialysis Center
& Hyperlipidemia Clinic

Barbara Delano, M.D., M.P.H.
Professor of Medicnine
Director, Home Hemodialysis & CAPD

Eli A. Friedman, M.D., M.A.C.P
Distinguished Teaching Professor of Med-
   icine
Chief, Renal Disease Division

Mariana Markell, M.D.
Associate Professor of Medicine
Director, Transplant Nephrology

Moro Salifu, M.D.
Assistant Professor of Medicine
Renal Disease Division

1. Correcting anemia slows renal disease progression

Eli A. Friedman

INTRODUCTION

Translating what is empirically established to a regimen designed to benefit an individual patient, in the absence of proof of efficacy, is the mainstay of medicine since its inception as a profession. Lacking evidence, but wanting to do good, is the rationale for "off label" extension of drugs as well as innovative though sometimes risky application of therapy.

Clinical "truths" are accepted without prospective, double-blind, placebo controlled trials. For example, few would dare question that penicillin alters the death rate in pneumococcal pneumonia though no studies meeting the above criteria have been reported. Further complicating the quest for new "hard" information is the ethical conundrum demanding appropriate controls. No Institutional Review Board would permit an alternate case trial of maintenance hemodialysis in which the "control" cohort received neither dialytic therapy nor a kidney transplant.

Similarly, testing the value of any new regimen for HIV infection cannot be done with a "no treatment control." Given the ethical constraints limiting contemporary investigation, what protocol might be employed to determine whether increasing the hematocrit by treatment with erythropoietin will slow the rate of renal functional loss?

Consensus interventions now applied

Listed in Table I are interventive measures reported to retard renal deterioration. Only the first two, normalizing hypertensive blood pressure and improving metabolic regulation in diabetes are established as effective by evidence based trials. In this context, how should the application of erythropoietin in anemic individuals with renal insufficiency who are not yet ready for uremia therapy be regarded?

Onyekachi Ifudu (ed.), Renal Anemia: Conflicts and Controversies, 1–7.
© *2002 Kluwer Academic Publishers.*

Table I. Measures that slow progressive renal disease [17]

1. Normalize hypertensive blood pressure [18]
2. Strive for euglycemia (diabetes) [19]
3. Limit dietary protein [20]
4. Restrict dietary lipids [21]
5. Reduce proteinuria [22]
6. Cease smoking [23]

Benefits of erythropoietin

As listed in Table II, there are irrefutable benefits of erythropoietin therapy in uremia. Evidence that erythropoietin is of clinical value in azotemia has been provided by Albertazzi and co-workers [1] who studied eighty-four pre-dialysis patients of mean age 61.7 ± 13.9 years, with hemoglobin levels between 6 and 9 g% and serum creatinine concentration ranging from 3 to 9 mg/dl who were treated with 2000 U of erythropoietin given subcutaneously twice weekly. After six months, mean hemoglobin increased from a baseline of 8.00 ± 0.77 g% to 10.06 ± 1.04 g%. Renal function, evaluated by plotting the reciprocal of serum creatinine values vs time, showed no impairment due to erythropoietin which was well tolerated, safe and effective.

That treatment with erythropoietin before dialysis confers a survival benefit to ESRD patients is evident in the analysis by Fink et al. [2] who reviewed records of the Health Care Financing Administration. When administered before the need for dialysis, of 4866 patients with a median follow-up was 26.2 months, the risk of death after starting dialysis was lower for patients treated with erythropoietin before dialysis compared with patients who were not treated (adjusted relative risk 0.80, 95% confidence interval 0.70 to 0.91). The most significant survival benefit attributed to erythropoietin use was in patients who attained the highest hematocrit values (adjusted relative risk 0.67, 95% confidence interval, 0.51 to 0.89).

Table II. Purported benefits of erythropoietin in irreversible renal failure [24]

1. Enhanced brain function [25]
2. Increased physical performance (endurance) [26]
3. Greatly improved quality of life [27]
4. Prevention of progressive left ventricular dilatation [28]
5. Elimination of blood transfusions [29]
6. Improved survival on hemodialysis/peritoneal dialysis [30,31]

A consensus case for erythropoietin therapy prior to initiation of ESRD therapy has grown sufficiently strong for Obrador et al. to characterize the circumstance of untreated anemia as suboptimal care [3]. Using data from Health Care Financing Administration these workers noted that at initiation of dialysis among 155,076 patients in the United States between April 1, 1995 and June 30, 1997, the median hematocrit was 28%, 51% had an hematocrit < 28%. Only 23% had received erythropoietin before development of ESRD. Interpreting the degree of discovered anemia to mean that pre-ESRD care in the United States requires attention, the authors speculate that "Improvement in pre-ESRD care could potentially improve outcomes among ESRD patients."

Table III. Potential value of erythropoietin pre-ESRD

---

1. Improves diabetic retinopathy (macular edema)
2. Decreases stress on left ventricle
3. Increases exercise tolerance
4. Decreases fatigue and somnolence
5. Enhances life quality
6. Delays progression of renal disease
7. Increases survival [32]

Erythropoietin in nephrosis

Erythropoietin deficiency accompanied normochromic normocytic anemia. The authors concluded that anemia associated with erythropoietin deficiency can occur early in diabetic nephropathy, but does not normally occur in nondiabetic renal disease of similar severity. Anemia, unresponsive to normalization of ferritin with iron treatment, is common the nephrotic syndrome in children whose renal function is normal.

In 19 nephrotic children who developed anemia before deterioration of kidney function, appropriate replacement therapy that normalized ferritin and/or cobalamin levels did not correct the anemia though the nephrotic children had higher levels of erythropoietin than did nephrotic children without anemia (21.6 ± 3.3 vs 5.5 ± 0.8 IU/L; $p < 0.001$). Treatment with erythropoietin in 6 of these 19 nephrotic children with hemoglobin levels less than 9 g/L corrected the anemia [4]. Underscoring the point that erythropoietin may be applicable in kidney disease when renal function is preserved are several case reports describing a similar rise in red cell mass in anemic nephrotic adults with intact renal function [5].

Table IV. Demonstrated efficacy of erythropoietin in anemic non-ESRD patients

1. Proteinuric type 1 diabetes
2. Nephrotic children with normal renal function
3. Nephrotic adults with normal renal function

Erythropoietin in diabetic nephropathy

Support for erythropoietin treatment early in the course of diabetic nephropathy is afforded by the report by Bosman et al. that of 27 proteinuric patients with type 1 diabetes, 13 were anemic (hemoglobin 10.6 ± 0.9 g/dl) compared with none of 26 proteinuric patients with glomerulonephritis (hemoglobin 13.7 ± 1.4 g/dl) and equivalent renal function (serum creatinine < or = 180 micromol/L) [6].

Additional benefits may accrue to anemic diabetic patients as erythropoietin slows the course of proliferative retinopathy [7] and macular edema [8]. Explaining these actions must be speculative as current empiric evidence is limited: it is known that diabetic individuals with mild nephropathy have reduced responsiveness (lower levels) of erythropoietin compared with other causes of kidney disease [9].

A single case report described a 52-year-old diabetic woman with proliferative retinopathy, autonomic neuropathy and microalbuminuria and moderate renal failure whose normochromic, normocytic aregenerative anaemia was associated with an inappropriately low concentration of erythropoietin [10]. Treatment with erythropoietin rapidly increased red cell mass and improved multiple diabetic complications.

Angiogeneis and hypoxia

Several angiogenesis factors have been proposed as responsible for vascular proliferation in the diabetic retina. Retinal ischemia induces intraocular neovascularization, promoting glaucoma, vitreous hemorrhage, and retinal detachment, presumably by stimulating the release of angiogenic molecules. An underlying hypothesis is that retinal microvasculopathy decreases retinal hypoperfusion and hypoxemia which in turn stimulates release of vascular growth factors from choroidal and other cells.

Angiogenin, for example, a potent blood vessel-inducing protein, was measured in undiluted vitreous fluid specimens collected at vitrectomy. In vitreous fluid from 21 patients with diabetic proliferative vitreoretinopathy the mean angiogenin level was 43.7 ng/ml, while in 21 control subjects with idiopathic macular epiretinal membrane mean concentration of angiogenin was 2.1 ng/ml [11]. These elevated angiogenin levels were interpreted as reflecting a breakdown of the blood-ocular barrier in proliferative diabetic retinopathy.

Altered retinal metabolism in diabetes has been linked to increased aldose reductase activity, hypoxia or "pseudohypoxia" (increase in NADH/NAD(+) attributed to increased sorbitol dehydrogenase activity). In streptozotocin-diabetic rats decreased mitochondrial and cytosolic NAD(+)/NADH ratios were completely or partially corrected by prazosin and DL-alpha-lipoic acid [12]. If hypoxia is the driving force resulting in diabetic eye disease [13], improving anemia may increase retinal oxygenation thereby blunting release of inducible growth factors that stimulate excess angiogenesis [14,15].

SUMMARY

Present consensus management of anemia in progressive renal insufficiency calls for correction of severe reduction in erythrocyte mass with erythropoietin while addressing other factors that might retard further renal injury (Table I). Undetermined, however, is a precise target level for an erythropoietin enabled hematocrit (hemoglobin), realizing that contingent on dose and frequency of administration, a return to normal and even erythrocythemia is readily attainable. Extrapolating from experience with maintenance hemodialysis and peritoneal dialysis, it appears an hematocrit of 35–38% optimizes well being, safe, and is cost effective [16]. Applying a regimen that has not reached the credibility of being evidence based forces a therapeutic gamble. On the proactive side, patients are subjected to a treatment that may be subsequently discredited as inefficacious or even injurious. The conservative "wait until proven" option may deny a helpful if not life-prolonging therapy to the present generation of patients.

For anemic individuals with nephrosis, pre-azotemic diabetic nephropathy, and/or progressive renal insufficiency, the downside risk of erythropoietin is nonexistent. Should subsequent prospective studies show that desire to retard renal disease is unattainable, the enhanced well being and improved exercise tolerance afforded by increased red cell mass is in itself a desirable end point.

REFERENCES

1. Albertazzi A, Di Liberato L, Daniele F, Battistel V, Colombi L. Efficacy and tolerability of recombinant human erythropoietin treatment in pre-dialysis patients: results of a multicenter study. Int J Artif Organs. 1998;21(1):12–8.
2. Fink J, Blahut S, Reddy M, Light P. Use of erythropoietin before the initiation of dialysis and its impact on mortality. Am J Kidney Dis. 2001;37(2):348–55.
3. Obrador GT, Ruthazer R, Arora P, Kausz AT, Pereira BJ. Prevalence of and factors associated with suboptimal care before initiation of dialysis in the United States. J Am Soc Nephrol. 1999;10(8):1793–800.
4. Feinstein S, Becker-Cohen R, Algur N, Raveh D, Shalev H, Shvil Y, Frishberg Y. Erythropoietin deficiency causes anemia in nephrotic children with normal kidney function. Am J Kidney Dis. 2001;37(4):736–42.
5. Ishimitsu T, Ono H, Sugiyama M, Asakawa H, Oka K, Numabe A, Abe M, Matsuoka H, Yagi S. Successful erythropoietin treatment for severe anemia in nephrotic syndrome without renal dysfunction. Nephron. 1996;74(3):607–10.
6. Bosman DR, Winkler AS, Marsden JT, Macdougall IC, Watkins PJ. Anemia with erythropoietin deficiency occurs early in diabetic nephropathy. Diabetes Care. 2001;24(3):495–9.
7. Berman DH, Friedman EA. Partial absorption of hard exudates in patients with diabetic end-stage renal disease and severe anemia after treatment with erythropoietin. Retina. 1994;14:1–5.
8. Friedman EA, Brown CD, Berman DH. Erythropoietin in diabetic macular edema and renal insufficiency. Am J Kidney Dis. 1995;26(1):202–8.
9. Yun YS, Lee HC, Yoo NC, Song YD, Lim SK, Kim KR, Hahn JS, Huh KB. Reduced erythropoietin responsiveness to anemia in diabetic patients before advanced diabetic nephropathy. Diabetes Res Clin Pract. 1999;46(3):223–9.
10. Hadjadj S, Torremocha F, Fanelli A, Brizard A, Bauwens M, Marechaud R. Erythropoietin-dependent anaemia: a possible complication of diabetic neuropathy. Diabetes Metab. 2001;27(3):383–5.
11. Ozaki H, Hayashi H, Oshima K. Angiogenin levels in the vitreous from patients with proliferative diabetic retinopathy. Ophthalmic Res. 1996;28:356–60.
12. Obrosova IG, Stevens MJ, Lang HJ. Diabetes-induced changes in retinal NAD-redox status pharmacological modulation and implications for pathogenesis of diabetic retinopathy. Pharmacology. 2001;62(3):172–80.
13. Kissun RD, Garner A. Vasoformative properties of normal and hypoxic retinal tissue. Br J Ophthalmol. 1977;61(6):394–8.
14. Miller JW, Adamis AP, Aiello LP. Vascular endothelial growth factor in ocular neovascularization and proliferative diabetic retinopathy. Diabetes Metab Rev. 1997;13(1):37–50.
15. Clermont AC, Aiello LP, Mori F, Aiello LM, Bursell SE. Vascular endothelial growth factor and severity of nonproliferative diabetic retinopathy mediate retinal hemodynamics in vivo: a potential role for vascular endothelial growth factor in the progression of nonproliferative diabetic retinopathy. Am J Ophthalmol. 1998;125:731–2.
16. Nissenson AR. Optimal hematocrit for hemodialysis. Curr Opin Nephrol Hypertens. 1997;6(6):524–7.
17. Basta E, Bakris GL.. Evolution of drugs that preserve renal function. J Clin Pharmacol. 2000;40:978–89.
18. Cinotti GA, Zucchelli PC. Collaborative Study Group. Effect of lisinopril on the progression of renal insufficiency in mild proteinuric non-diabetic nephropathies. Nephrol Dial Transplant. 2001;16(5):961–6.

19. Chase HP, Lockspeiser T, Peery B, Shepherd M, MacKenzie T, Anderson J, Garg SK. The impact of the diabetes control and complications trial and humalog insulin on glycohemoglobin levels and severe hypoglycemia in type 1 diabetes. Diabetes Care. 2001;24(3):430–4.
20. Fouque D, Wang P, Laville M, Boissel JP. Low protein diets for chronic renal failure in non diabetic adults (Cochrane Review). Cochrane Database Syst Rev. 2001;2:CD001892.
21. Schmitz PG. Progressive renal insufficiency. Office strategies to prevent or slow progression of kidney disease. Postgrad Med. 2000;108(1):145–8, 151–4.
22. Keane WF. Proteinuria: its clinical importance and role in progressive renal disease. Am J Kidney Dis. 2000;35(4 supplement 1):S97–105.
23. Righetti M, Sessa A. Cigarette smoking and kidney involvement. J Nephrol. 2001;14(1):3–6.
24. Murphy ST, Parfrey PS. Erythropoietin therapy in chronic uremia: the impact of normalization of hematocrit. Curr Opin Nephrol Hypertens. 1999;8(5):573–8.
25. Macdougall IC. Quality of life and anemia: the nephrology experience. Semin Oncol. 1998;25(3 supplement 7):39–42.
26. Johansen KL. Physical functioning and exercise capacity in patients on dialysis. Adv Ren Replace Ther. 1999;6(2):141–8.
27. Brandberg Y. Quality of life in clinical trials: assessment and utility with special reference to rHuEPO. Med Oncol. 1998;15(supplement 1):S8–12.
28. McMahon LP, Mason K, Skinner SL, Burge CM, Grigg LE, Becker GJ. Effects of haemoglobin normalization on quality of life and cardiovascular parameters in end-stage renal failure. Nephrol Dial Transplant. 2000;15:1425–30.
29. Page DE, House A. Important cost differences of blood transfusions and erythropoietin between hemodialysis and peritoneal dialysis patients. Adv Perit Dial. 1998;14:87–9.
30. Mocks J. Cardiovascular mortality in haemodialysis patients treated with epoetin beta – a retrospective study. Nephron. 2000;86(4):455–62.
31. Collins AJ, Ma JZ, Ebben J. Impact of hematocrit on morbidity and mortality. Semin Nephrol. 2000;20(4):345–9.
32. Macdougall IC. How to improve survival in pre-dialysis patients. Nephron 2000;85(supplement 1):15–22.

2. Does treatment with EPO improve RBC survival ?

Clinton D. Brown, Zhong H. Zhao, Lorraine L. Thomas, Robert deGroof and Eli A. Friedman

INTRODUCTION

Anemia is a common complication of acute and chronic renal failure and prior to the onset of ESRD, it is a usual clinical feature of renal insufficiency. Correction of the anemia associated with renal disease by erythropoietin (EPO) treatment, has proven to be a major contribution to the general medical care of patients with renal failure. Aside from clinically significant improvement in hematocrit, EPO treatment has resulted in significant improvement in physical working capacity, appetite, physical well-being [1], cognitive performance [2], and sexual function [3].

EPO regulates the production of erythrocytes by preventing apoptosis (programmed death) of intramarrow late erythroid progenitor cells (survival factor) [4] and there is evidence that EPO also functions as a mitogen for early erythroid progenitor [5]. The topic that will be explored in this article is whether EPO has an effect on the vitality of RBCs [in circulation] in patients with renal disease. As suggested by Zachee et al. [6], uremic toxin(s) may play a significant role in renal associated anemia. In a previous experiment, RBCs taken from normal volunteers and infused into uremic patients have significantly shortened survival. Conversely, RBC survival is restored to normal when RBCs from uremic patients are infused into normal subjects [7].

Advanced glycation end products – A uremic toxin

Advanced glycation end products (AGEs) are a heterogeneous group of highly reactive carbonyl compounds formed on proteins and peptides by nonenzymatic glycation and or glycoxidation. AGEs accumulate in tissues

Onyekachi Ifudu (ed.), Renal Anemia: Conflicts and Controversies, 9–13.
© 2002 *Kluwer Academic Publishers.*

over time as part of normal aging. However, their rate of production, tissue and plasma accumulation are markedly accelerated in diabetes and in renal disease. AGE formation results in alteration in protein function and or structure, and is thought to play a role in causing late complication of diabetes [8].

There is occurring evidence that AGEs are uremic toxins. Levels of AGE have been shown to correlate with renal impairment [9,10]. In addition AGEs have been shown to modify dialysis related β_2-microglobulin-amyloid [11], and contribute to the development of atherosclerosis [12] in patients with ESRD regardless of the presence or absence of diabetes. Furthermore, it has been shown that 3-deoxyglucosone, an AGE precursor and product of the Maillard reaction, inhibits RBC antioxidant enzymes, glutathione peroxidase and glutathione reductase [13]. This action may further cause injury to the RBC and enhance oxidative stress in patients with ESRD.

RBC deformability and RBC survival in renal failure

Normally, as the circulating RBC matures there is a progressive loss in its ability to deform. Older and less deformable cells are selectively removed by the reticulum endothelial system. Using a 5 micron pore filtration system to measure RBC-df, Zachee et al. [6] and Macdugall et al. [14] have shown that impaired RBC- df in patients with ESRD (on hemodialysis) was not improved by treatment with EPO despite improvement in hematocrit. It was concluded [6] that failure of correction in impaired RBC-df supports previous reports [15,16] of reduced RBC life span in uremic patients on hemodialysis.

In two controlled trials of EPO, treatment in dialysis patients [17,18] in which RBC survival was measured using the chromium 51 technique, it found that EPO treatment resulted in significant improvement the life span of the RBC. In the study by Polenakovic and Sikole [17], RBC survival was measured at baseline (pre-EPO), one year during EPO treatment and one year after EPO was discontinued. During EPO treatment RBC survival was improved to just below the normal range. In contrast, RBC survival reverted to baseline (no EPO) levels one year after EPO was discontinued. These data suggest that EPO has a positive effect the longevity of RBCs in uremic patients on dialysis.

In contrast to the reports of Zachee [6] and Macdugall [14], we have reported that EPO significantly improves RBC-df in diabetic patients with renal insufficiency (pre-dialysis) after 6 months of treatment. This effect was sustained for twelve months despite progression in renal disease [19].

In our study we used a 3 micron pore filter to measure RBC-df which may explain why our findings were different from that of Zachee [6] and Macdugall [14] who used a larger 5 micron pore filter. In our experience the 3 micron pore filter is a better detector of subtle differences in RBC-df.

We previously reported that impaired RBC-df measured in the induced hyperglycemic rabbit may be linked to AGEs [20]. In that study, amino-guanidine, a potent inhibitor of AGEs given by oral gavage to alloxan induced-diabetic rabbits for 12 weeks restored RBC-df to normal. Conversely, RBC-df deteriorated and returned to the pre-treatment impairment 10 weeks after aminoguanidine was withdrawn. In a collateral study from our group, we found that treatment with aminoguanidine in diabetic dialysis patients on a stable dose of EPO, significantly improved RBC-df to near normal [19]. EPO is not a known inhibitor of AGEs and AGEs are maximally elevated in all patients with ESRD regardless of the patient's glycemic status. What then might be a plausible mechanism through which EPO might impact favorable on RBC-df and RBC survival?

The answer to this is not known. However we propose three reasonable possibilities. First, EPO treatment may result in the generation of a highly deformable RBC. Secondly, it is known that EPO treatment in dialysis patients results significant improvement in protein catabolism [21]. This may be important since reduction in the breakdown of protein stores could result in diminished release of AGE-peptides into the circulation. Finally, low molecular Plasma AGEs are cleared, though transiently, with each dialytic treatment. The amount of AGEs cleared per dialysis depends on the dialyzer used (for example, from 22% to 84% reduction have been reported [22]). It is conceivable that the combination of these three events (generation of highly deformable RBC, stabilization of protein metabolism, intermittent removal of low molecular weight AGES) occurring over a prolonged period (> 1 year) might significantly improve the longevity of the RBC in patients on maintenance hemodialysis.

REFERENCES

1.   Eshbach JW, Egrie JC, Downing MR, Brown JK, Adamson JW. Correction of the anemia of end-stage renal disease with recombinant human erythropoietin. N Engl J Med. 1987;316:73–8.

2. Nissenson AR, Marsh JT, Brown WS, Schweitzer S, Wolcott DL. Brain function improves in chronic hemodialysis patients after recombinant erythropoietin. Kidney Int. 1989;35:25.

3. Bommer J, Alexiou C, Muller-Buhl U, Eifery J, Ritz E. Recombinant human erythropoietin therapy in heamodiallysis patients – dose determination and clinical experience. Nephrol Dial Transplantation. 1987;2:238–42.

4. Mark J, Bondurant MC. Erythropoietin retards DAN breakdown and prevents programmed death in erythroid progenitor cells. Science. 1990;248:376–81.

5. Spivak JL, Pham T, Isaacs M, Hankins D. Erythropoietin is both a mitogen and a survival factor. Blood. 1991;177:1228–33.

6. Zachee P, Ferrant A, Daelemans R, Coolen L, Goossens W, Lins RL, Coutteye X, De Broe ME, Boogaerts MA. Oxidative injury to erythrocytes, cell rigidity and splenic hemolysis in hemodialyzed patients before and during erythropoietin treatment. Nephron. 1993;65:288–93.

7. Joske RA, McAlister JM, Prankert TAJ. Isotope investigations of red cell production and destruction in chronic renal disease. Clin Sci. 1956;15:511–22.

8. William SK, Howarth NL, Devenny JS, Bitensky MW. Structural and functional consequences of increased tubulin glycosylation in diabetes mellitus. Proc Natl Acad Sci USA. 1982;79:6546–50.

9. Weiss MP, Rodby AR, Justice AC, Hricik DE and The Colavorative Study Group. Free pentosidine and neopterin as markers of progression rate in diabetic nephropathy. Kidney Int. 1998;54:193–202.

10. Sebekova K, Blakzick P, Syrova D, Krivosikova Z, Soustova V, Heidland A, Schinzel R. Circulating advanced glycation end product level in rats rapidly increase with acute renal failure. Kidney Int. 2001;78:S58–S62.

11. Capeillere-Blandin C, Delaveau T, Descamps-Latxha B. Structural modification of human B2 microglobulin treated with oxygen-derived radicals. Biochem J. 1991; 277:175–82.

12. Vlassara H. Advanced location end-products atherosclerosis. Ann Int Med. 1996; 28:419–26.

13. Niwa T, Tsukushi S. 3-Deoxyglucosone and AGEs in uremic complications: inactivation of glutathione peroxidase by 3-deoxyglucosone. Kidney Int. 2001; 78:S37–S41.

14. Macdugall IC, Davies ME, Hutton RD, Coles GA, Williams JD. Rheological studies during treatment of renal anemias with recombinant human erythropoietin. Br J Hematol. 1991;77:550–8.

15. Zender C, Blumberg A. Human recombinant erythropoietin treatment in transfusion dependent anemic patient on maintenance hemodialysis. Clin Nephrol. 1989;31:55–9.

16. Cotes PM, Pippaard MJ, Reid CDL, Winearls CG, Oliver DO, Royston JP. Characterization of anemia of chronic renal failure and the mode of its correction by a preparation of human erythropoietin. An investigation of the pharmacokinetics of intravenous erythropoietin and its effect on erythrokinetics. QJ Med. 1989;7:113–37.

17. Polenakovic M, Sikole A. Is erythropoietin a survival factor for red blood cells? J Am Soc Nephrol. 1996;7:1178–82.

18. Schwartz AB, Kahn SB, Kelch B, Kim KE, Pequignot E. RBC improved survival due to recombinant human erythropoietin explains effectiveness of less frequent, low dose subcutaneous therapy. Clin Nephrol. 1992;38:283–9.

19. Brown CD, Zhao ZH, Thomas LL, deGroof R, Friedman EA. Effects of erythropoietin and aminoguanidine of red blood cell deformability in diabetic azotemic and uremic patients. Am J Kid Dis. (in press).

20. Brown CD, Zhao ZH, DeAlvaro F, Chan S, Friedman EA. Correction of erythrocyte deformability defect in ALX-induced diabetic rabbits after treatment with aminoguanidine. Diabetes. 1993;16:590–3.
21. Fischer C, Scigalla P, Park W, Becker H, Schiller R, Paust H, Broesicke H, Kessel M. influence of rhEPO therapy on the protein metabolism of hemodialysis patients with terminal renal insufficiency. Contrib Nephrol. 1989;76;250–6.
22. Nicl T, Lapolla A, Arico CN, Gammaro L, Bernich P, Fedele D. Hemodialysis techniques and advanced glycation end products. Contrib Nephrol. 2001;131: 33–9.

3. Has the best route of administration for epoetin been established?

Anatole Besarab and Rebecca Schmidt

INTRODUCTION

The best route for administration of erythropoietin in patients with end stage renal disease (ESRD) continues to spark debate. In the USA, the intravenous (IV) route is most widely used, mostly for convenience, despite the demonstration that total weekly dose to achieve/maintain a given target hemoglobin (Hb) level is lower with subcutaneously (SC) administered erythropoietin [1]. The interplay between dose, efficacy, acquisition cost, and revenue generation engages prioritization of both known factors physiology of erythropoiesis, pharmacokinetics of erythropoiesis, desired target hemoglobin, dose size effect, underlying illnesses – and uncertain factors, such as the optimal (best) target hemoglobin and each individual patient's physiologic response.

Despite guidelines set forth by the Dialysis Outcomes Quality Initiative in 1997 [2] recommending the SC route for recombinant human erythropoietin (rHuEPO) administration, the majority of ESRD patients in the United States receive rHuEPO by intravenously rather than SC (90% vs. 10%) [3]. The European Best Practice Guidelines for anemia management also advocate the SC route [4], and in Europe IV administration is more common than SC even though the goals of anemia management are virtually the same.

Numerous studies conducted over the last decade have attempted to quantify and compare the efficacy of IV and SC administration of rHuEPO in patients with renal anemia [5–14]. Opposition to the "superiority" of the SC route, if efficacy is quantitated as the increase in Hb achieved divided by the epoetin dose used, centered on the small samples in the studies, methodological differences among them, and differences in treatment duration and dosing strategy. However, the VAH co-operative study clearly

Onyekachi Ifudu (ed.), Renal Anemia: Conflicts and Controversies, 15–28.
© 2002 *Kluwer Academic Publishers.*

showed that on average the SC route was more efficacious [1]. In this study, despite potential other confounding factors, such as patient variability in subcutaneous absorption and functional iron depletion, average epoetin dose needed to maintain the same target Hb was 35% lower with the SC than with the IV route. Thus with the current formulation of the unmodified rHuEPO molecule, the bulk of evidence supports the SC route as the most efficacious because it produces sustained blood levels that minimize apoptosis during normal erythropoiesis [8]. However, this may change as modifications to the molecule are made or alternative means of delivery are developed.

The concept of apoptosis is key with regard to clinical dosing practices. The optimal dosing regimen is one that prevents this process. It's importance can only be understood by a consideration of erythropoiesis and its dependence on concentration-time profiles. Preventing apoptosis to optimize the bone marrow response is central to the development of more "efficient" epoetins.

Erythropoiesis

In the normal physiologic steady state, plasma levels of erythropoietin in a given individual are remarkably constant. Renal response to severe anemia in normal subjects can result in a 100–1000 fold increase in kidney erythropoietin production (Figure 1). By contrast, maximum response of the bone marrow is limited to only a 4–6 fold increase in erythrocyte production [15]. Diseased kidneys can augment transiently their EPO production in response to an appropriate anemic hypoxic stimulus such as blood loss [16] but the plasma levels achieved are still lower than those achieved by normal individuals who sustain an equivalent degrees of blood loss.

Overall there is a shift down and to the right in the dose response curve (Figure 1) in patients with advanced Chronic Kidney Disease (CKD) or on dialysis. Under conditions in which increased red cell production is required, the kidney augments and sustains the plasma levels of erythro-poiesis.

Since the major biologic effect of erythropoietin is to regulate the number of committed erythroid precursors and promote maturation into erythrocytes (Figure 2), the *constant presence of erythropoietin* is critical to the sustenance, multiplication, and differentiation of committed erythroid progenitors. To achieve the same degree of red cell production, the erythropoietin level must be about 5–8 times higher in patients with CKD than in normal subjects (40–150 mU/ml vs. 4–24 mU/ml).

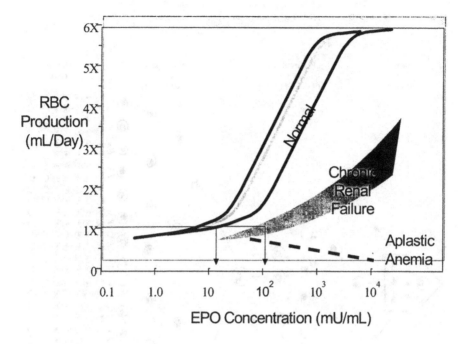

Figure 1. Erythropoietic dose responses in normals and those with advanced chronic kidney disease (CKD). There is a shift down and to the right in CKD (creatinine > 4 mg/dl or dialysis). In order to maintain a normal rate of red blood cells, plasma levels in CKD, must be maintained approximately 5–8 times higher than in normal subjects

Cells differentiating under the influence of erythropoietin undergo apoptosis and die if the EPO levels decrease below a critical level needed to maintain them throughout maturation (Figure 2). The appearance of erythroid receptors on burst-forming units-erythroid (BFU-E) correlates with the onset of erythropoietin dependency. At the BFU-E and colony-forming units-erythroid (CFU-E) stages, erythropoietin not only amplifies the number of cells but also promotes their survival.

Within the BFU-E compartment, sensitivity to erythropoietin increases with increasing cellular maturation. The CFU-E is the most sensitive to and dependent on erythropoietin and has the largest number of receptors. At a certain level of maturation the CFU-E becomes activated and the cells are transformed into hemoglobin synthesizing morphologically recognizable erythroblasts (Figure 1). Receptor density decreases at the proerythroblast and erythroblast stage and the reticulocyte apparently has no detectable receptors.

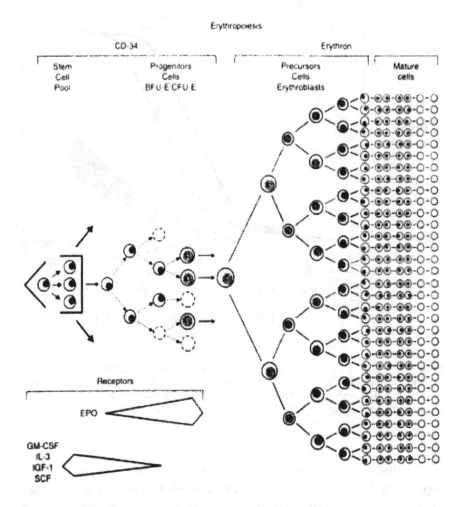

Figure 2. Differentiation and maturation of red blood cells. EPO receptors develop in the BFU-E and CFU-E stages and receptor density increases. Absence of epoetin during this stage of maturation leads to apoptosis (ghosts). Once cells leave the CFU-E and become erythroblasts, they can become reticulocytes. Each epoetin-independent cell produces 32 mature cells

Further proliferation and maturation of these cells appear to be unaffected by erythropoietin and proceeds at a fixed rate in the presence of adequate supplies of iron, folate, vitamin B12, pyridoxine, ascorbic acid, and trace elements. The total duration during which CFU and CFU cells are absolutely dependent on epoetin is approximately 3–5 days.

Pharmacokinetics and pharmacodynamics

High epoetin peak levels followed by rapid decline, as occurs following IV administration, produce a state conducive to apoptosis since the development of increasing numbers of receptors on CFU-E requires more rather than less epoetin to be available. It takes less erythropoietin to start the process than to sustain it. The time profile following IV administration is the exact opposite of that required. Indeed, thirty years ago, crude preparations of erythropoietin administered in small portions produced a greater effect on red cell production than when the erythropoietin was given all at once [17,18].

Even then it was understood that the erythropoietic response was not dependent on the peak concentration of erythropoietin but on the duration of time that erythropoietin levels were maintained above a critical concentration. The corresponding pharmacokinetic term is mean residence time.

It seems logical therefore that a continuous rather than intermittent stimulus would better mimic the conditions required to induce the appropriate bone marrow response as typically occurs with normal renal function. Currently, there are no reliable and practical methods by which sustained epoetin levels can be achieved using the first generation rHuEPO formulations. Rather the route and frequency of administration determine the concentration-time profiles achieved.

Differences in temporal profile IV vs. SC

Early trials of EPO to patients with renal failure were done without background knowledge as to the optimal dose or route of administration. IV administration was utilized in order to ensure that 100% of the exogenously supplied EPO was sufficient to stimulate the bone marrow and erythropoiesis. Subsequent pharmacokinetic studies suggested that SC administration provided a dose advantage, hence the start of an ongoing debate challenging the unproven superiority of IV over SC.

Initial clinical trials focused on the thrice-weekly intravenous administration of EPO in ESRD patients on hemodialysis, the efficacy of the intravenous route assumed. Comparison studies conducted over the last decade have led many leading authorities to champion the use of SC epoetin administration over IV, though with some caveats. The majority of these studies [1,5–10] suggest a dose-for-dose superiority of the SC route over IV, and results of several [9,10] suggest that not only is the dose required to reach target lower with SC, but that the time required to reach a maintenance dose is shorter as well. The most convincing of these studies is that of Kaufmann et al. [1] who performed a randomized clinical trial within the VAH system. A minority of investigators [11–14] have reported equivalent results with IV and SC. There is no data to suggest that SC is inferior to IV for epoetin administration. From a purely efficacy point of view, the SC route delivers more "bang for the buck" and when health resources are limited, it is the rational route for administration.

The pharmacodynamic advantage of the SC route derives from its pharmacokinetic profile. The temporal profile of subcutaneously administered EPO differs from that administered intravenously [8,19–24]. In general, the bioavailability following subcutaneous administration is much less than that following an equal intravenous dose, shows a very large inter-patient variability, and the time to maximum concentration is delayed beyond 10 hours (Figure 3).

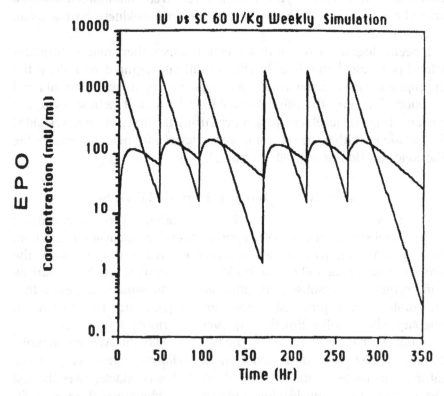

Figure 3. Comparison of epoetin concentration profiles following equivalent doses administered IV and SC. Concentrations are increments above baseline. Based on the pharmacokinetic data in reference 8. Note the very low epoetin concentrations particularly in the 3-day dosing interval following IV but not SC administration. If maintenance levels > 50 mU/ml are needed to avoid apoptosis, then larger amounts of epoetin must be administered IV

Although the maximum concentration achieved by a given dose following subcutaneous administration is frequently only 10% of that seen after intravenous dosing, adequate plasma levels are maintained for a prolonged period permitting some accumulation of EPO level if the dosing interval is 48 hours or less (vida infra). Our pharmacokinetic studies [8] and those of others indicate that the pharmacokinetic profiles do not change after a year or more of treatment [25].

The average half-life of eythropoietin (about 6–8 hours) is relatively short compared to the usual dosing interval (44 to 68 hours). When given intravenously, although peak epoetin levels can exceed 1000 mU/ml (normal levels 4–24 mU/ml), the blood levels are not sustained and the mean residence time is low. By contrast, following SC dosing, more consistent and sustained levels are achieved (Figure 3). The more gradual but more sustained concentration levels seen following SC administrations can prevent the inefficient erythropoiesis associated with apoptosis.

Hence, the erythropoietic response is not dependent on the peak concentration of erythropoietin achieved but on the duration of time that erythropoietin levels are maintained above a critical concentration. Even more constant epoetin levels can be obtained by administering the epoetin more frequently, i.e., daily, and this reduces the dose needed to achieve a target Hb [26]. In one study, a continuous subcutaneous infusion of EPO in malnourished predialysis patients with diabetic nephropathy increased Hb by 2.6 g/dl within 4 weeks while EPO levels increased from 18 and were maintained at 75 mU/ml. The same weekly EPO dose (6000 IU) given as a single subcutaneous injection had no effect on Hb nor on reticulocyte count [27].

The route and frequency for EPO administration clearly influences the plasma concentration-time profiles. Which route to use is likely to change in the next few years as methods are developed that change the pharmacokinetic properties of the hormone and its possible administration. Certainly as the need to attain or sustain higher Hb levels become apparent, some centers decreased their use of the SC route as doses increased and larger volumes had to be injected, particularly in those patients manifesting a hyporesponse to therapy.

Target levels

Over the past decade the target Hb has changed (Figure 4). Both the desired (optimal) Hb level as well as its clinical counterpart, the achieved Hb have increased. For patients with ESRD, administration of rHuEPO dosed to achieve a target Hb of 11–12.5 gm/dl (or hematocrit (Hct) of 33–

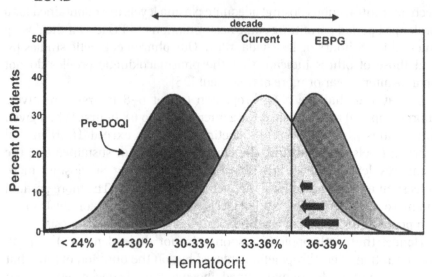

DISTRIBUTION CURVES FOR ANEMIA MANAGEMENT - ESRD

Figure 4. Over the past decade, the mean Hb of ESRD recipients in the United States has increased from less than 10 g/dl to about 11.6 g/dl. This has occurred in response to the DOQI guidelines. The arrows indicate the need to prevent the Hb from exceeding 12.5 g/dl on a 3-month rolling average in order to receive payments. The European Best Practice Guidelines (EBPG) do not have an absolute upper limit and their distribution can shift to the right

36%) is standard of care and as well as being the range within which Medicare reimbursement is allowed. The optimal hematocrit during EPO therapy in ESRD patients is currently unknown, although the failed "normal hematocrit trial" [28], NKF-DOQI guidelines [2], and recent analyses of US ESRD mortality [29] suggest that a target hemoglobin of 11–13 g/dl maximizes benefit and minimizes morbidity. The rHuEPO dose can be increased to achieve any level of hemoglobin. The real challenge is to determine the optimal hemoglobin in a specific patient and the best route for that patient. Unfortunately getting the patient to the target Hb and the best route for keeping the patient at target Hb is confounded by the following.

Response variability

Variability may be the operative word. Thrice-weekly maintenance intravenous doses needed to maintain steady state Hb between 11–12 g/dl are quite variable among patients, from less than a 1000 U per treatment to over a 10,000 U [30–32]. In part this variability reflects the observation that even in normal individuals, a 10-fold variability in endogenous erythropoietin levels among subjects evidently maintains the same normal red cell mass [30].

This variation in EPO levels suggests that significant differences in bone marrow sensitivity exist among individuals to erythropoietin. Wide variability in the dose-response of the bone marrow to erythropoietin has prompted the use of different dosing strategies: initiation at low doses (20 U/kg subcutaneously), gradual increase to obtain the desired response [33] vs. initiation with thrice weekly intravenous doses of $\geqslant 100$ U/kg [34].

The sensitivity of a given patient to exogenous EPO is unknown at the beginning of therapy, hence it is difficult to predict a dose of erythropoietin required by an individual patient to initiate and maintain effective erythropoiesis. Failed kidneys continue to produce erythropoietin though the amount produced is much less than that required and the levels achieved, while inappropriately low [35,36], may also influence exogenous dose requirement.

Other confounders

The difficulty inherent in comparing route of administration studies, which employ different methods, dosing strategies and treatment times has been confounded by the recognition that individual patients respond differently to both IV and SC administered EPO. A wide interpatient variability in the response to both SC and IV EPO has been noted by several investigators, who caution that SC administration may not be better than IV in every patient. This finding is well illustrated by Barclay et al. [11] who conducted a double crossover study of 10 hemodialysis patients receiving IV, followed by SC, and a second period of IV rHEPO. Higher hemoglobins were not exclusively associated with administration of IV and SC rHuEPO; in fact, some patients had their highest Hb levels when receiving EPO IV, suggesting that the most efficient route of administration for a particular patient cannot be predicted.

A multi-center study [1] comparing IV and SC dosing using a crossover design in a study of 108 hemodialysis patients provides further evidence for wide variety of patient responses, albeit at lower weekly doses. In 61%

of these study patients, doses were reduced following the switch from IV to SC. The remaining 39% required the same or greater doses of rHuEPO, underscoring the variability inherent in patient response [1].

Current recommendations

The ESRD Core Indicators Work Group, in an attempt to reconcile the divergence between DOQI recommended guidelines and actual clinical practice, recently analyzed hematocrit levels in nearly 7000 ESRD patients receiving exogenous erythropoietin [3]. Results from this analysis suggest that in actual clinical practice, the dose of subcutaneously administered rHuEPO being used to achieve target hemoglobin is clearly less than that required when give intravenously. These findings are consistent with the abundance of evidence from clinical trials that led to the DOQI recommendations advocating the use of subcutaneous EPO. Based on these parallel findings, the work group encourages physicians to consider the subcutaneous route of EPO administration in dialysis patients.

The pharmacokinetic and pharmacodynamic profile observed following subcutaneous administration [8] suggest that cost-benefit is achieved by maintenance of sustained erythropoietin levels within a critical range (about 40–150 mU/ml above basal) following subcutaneous rather than on very high transient but less sustained levels following intravenous administration. For normal as well as renal failure patients, we [8] and others [5,13,30,37] have shown that subcutaneous administration of rHuEPO produces a more favorable pharmacodynamic effect than intravenous administration. If cost-effectiveness of therapy is expressed as the increment in hemoglobin achieved (benefit) per unit dose of EPO (cost) used, then more effective erythropoiesis requires more and not lesser frequencies of administration. Administering even smaller doses once a day subcutaneously produces the most efficient response and requires the smallest total weekly dose [36,38].

On the horizon

Modification of the parent hormone and development of alternate delivery systems are under active investigation. The goal is to produce sustained elevations in plasma levels to minimize ineffective erythropoiesis secondary to cell death. Recently approved for use in renal anemia, the novel erythropoietic stimulating substance (NESP), is a modification of the native hormone that results in a prolongation of elimination constant following IV administration (Figure 5) [39]. Preliminary results suggest

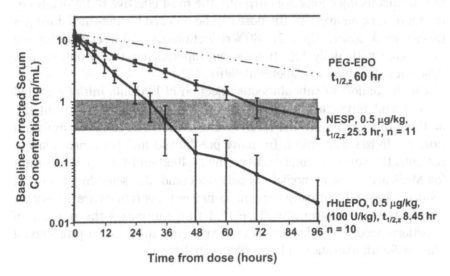

Figure 5. Prolonging the biological action of epoetin by modification. (Adapted from Reference 39)

that its prolonged circulation time will permit dosing intervals to be increased in many patients (one a week dosing in hemodialysis is possible, personal observations). However, when NESP is given SC, adequate levels are sustained for over a week making it the possible to dose patients with CKD or on peritoneal dialysis as infrequently as every 2–3 weeks.

Even longer sustenance of the circulating hormone is possible by attaching the molecule to a carrier such as polyethylene glycol. This PEG-EPO is reported to have a half-life of 60 hours. Whether it can be administered SC is currently unknown.

As these preparations are developed and transcutaneous methods are developed to permit sustained maintenance of blood levels, the argument as to which route is optimal is likely to become moot. It will then be a question of the setting, i.e., anemia in the pre dialysis period, which in some cases can last for years, availability of an intravenous route to avoid pain, the target hemoglobin that is to be achieved or maintained.

CONCLUSIONS

Subcutaneous injections are currently the most effective route of administration since on average, the dose can be reduced by one-third during 3 times a week dosing. Up to 70–80% reductions in total weekly dosing are achievable with daily injections if one approaches the situation as a deficiency state akin to diabetes mellitus.

The discomfort of subcutaneous injection of EPO alfa initially limited patient and physician acceptance of the subcutaneous route but the addition of a benzyl alcohol (preservative/anesthetic) to the formulation now minimizes discomfort. In many pre-dialysis and peritoneal dialysis patients, the subcutaneous route permits self-administration. Were it not for Medicare rules, hemodialysis patients could also self-administer and reduce some of the nursing burden. As newer preparations are developed, clearly the optimal route will be that that minimizes the number of injections needed, the discomfort to the patients, the need for professional staff (self-administration at home just as in diabetes)

REFERENCES

1. Kaufman JS, Reda DJ, Fye CI, Goldfarb DS, Henderson WG, Kleinmann JG, Vaamonde CA. Subcutaneous compared to intravenous epoetin in patients receiving hemodialysis. Department of Veterans Affairs Cooperative Study Group on Erythropoietin in Hemo-dialysis patients. N Engl J Med .1998;339:578–83.

2. National Kidney Foundation-Dialysis Outcomes Quality Initiative. NKF-DOQI clinical practice guidelines for the treatment of anemia of chronic renal failure. Am J Kidney Dis. 1997;30:S192–240.

3. McClellan WM, Frankenfield DL, Wish JB, Rocco MV, Johnson CA, Owen WF, for the End-Stage Renal Disease Core Indicators Work Group. Subcutaneous erythropoietin results in lower dose and equivalent hematocrit levels among adult hemodialysis patients: results from the 1998 end-stage renal disease core indicators project. Am J Kidney Dis. 2001;37(5);E36.

4. Jacobs C, Horl WH, Macdougall IC, Valderrabano F, Parrondo I, Abraham IL, Segner A. European best practice guidelines 9–13 anaemia management. Nephrol Dial Transplantation. 2000;15(supplement 4):33–42.

5. Albitar S, Meulders Q, Hammoud H, Soutif C, Bouvier P, Pollini J. Sub-cutaneous versus intravenous administration of erythropoietin improves its efficiency for the treatment of anaemia in haemodialysis patients. Nephrol Dial Transplantation. 1995;10(supplement 6):40–3.

6. Paganini EP, Eschbach JW, Lazarus JM, Van Stone JC, Gimenez LF, Graber SE, Egrie JC, Okamoto DM, Goodkin DA. Intravenous versus subcutaneous dosing of epoetin alfa in hemodialysis patients. Am J Kidney Dis. 1995;26(2):331–40.

7. Tomson CRV, Feehally J, Walls J. Crossover comparison of intravenous and subcutaneous erythropoietin in haemodialysis patients. Nephrol Dial Transplantation. 1992;7:129–32.

8. Besarab A, Flaharty KK, Erslev AJ, et al. Clinical Pharmacology and economics of recombinant human erythropoietin in end-stage renal disease: the case for subcutaneous administration. J Am Soc Nephrol. 1992;2:1405–16.

9. Eidemak I, Friedberg MO, Ladefoged SD, Lokkegaard H, Pedersen E, Skielboe M. Intra-venous versus subcutaneous administration of recombinant human erythropoietin in patients on haemodialysis and CAPD. Nephrol Dial Transplantation 1992;7:526–9.

10. Muirhead N, Churchill DN, Goldstein M, Nadler SP, Posen G, Wong C, Slaughter D, Laplante P. Comparison of subcutaneous and intravenous recombinant human erythropoietin for anemia in hemodialysis patients with significant comorbid disease. Am J Nephrol. 1992;12:303–10.

11. Barclay PG, Fischer ER, Harris DCH. Interpatient variation in response to subcutaneous versus intravenous low dose erythropoietin. Clin Nephrol. 1993; 40(5):277–80.

12. Schaller R, Sperschneider H, Thieler H, Dutz W, Hans S, Voigt D, Marx M, Engelmann J, Schoter K-H, Scigalla P, Stein G. Differences in intravenous and subcutaneous application of recombinant human erythropoietin: a multicenter trial. Artif Organ. 1994;18(8):552–8.

13. Parker KP, Mitch WE, Stivelman JC, Macon EJ, Bailey JL, Sands JM. Safety and efficacy of low-dose subcutaneous erythropoietin in hemodialysis patients. J Am Soc Nephrol. 1997;8:288–93.

14. Jensen JD, Madsen JK, Jensen LW. Comparison of dose requirement, serum erythropoietin and blood pressure following intravenous and subcutaneous erythropoietin treatment of dialysis patients. Eur J Clin Pharmacol. 1996;50: 171–7.

15. Erslev AJ. Erythropoietin. N Engl J Med. 1991;324:1339–44.

16. Ross R, McCrea JB, Besarab A. Erythropoietin response to blood loss in hemodialysis patients in blunted but preserved. ASAIO J. 1994;40:M880–5.

17. Fogh J. The increased dose response of ESF after ESF stimulation. Ann NY Acad Sci. 1968;149:217–22.

18. Gurney CW, Wackman N, Filmanowitz E. Studies on erythropoiesis. XVII. Some quantitative aspects of the erythropoietic response to erythropoietin. Blood. 1961;17:531–46.

19. Veng-Pendersen P, Widness JA, Pereira LM, Peters C, Schmidt RL, Lowe LS. Kinetic evaluation of nonlinear drug elimination by a disposition decomposition analysis. Application to the analysis of the nonlinear elimination kinetics of erythropoietin in adult humans. J Pharm Sci. 1995;84:760–7.

20. McMahon FG, Vargas R, Ryan M, Jain AK, Abels RI, Smith PB, Smith IL. Pharmacokinetics and effects of recombinant human erythropoietin after intravenous and subcutaneous injections in healthy volunteers. Blood. 1990;76: 1718–22.

21. Hughes RT, Cotes PM, Oliver DO, et al. Correction of anemia of chronic renal failure with erythropoietin: pharmacokinetic studies in patients on hemodialysis and CAPD. Contrib Nephrol. 1989;76:122–30.

22. Salmonson T. Pharmacokinetic and pharmacodynamic studies on recombinant human erythropoietin. Scand J Urol Nephrol. 1990;129(supplement):1–66.

23. Nielsen OJ. Pharmacokinetics of recombinant human erythropoietin in chronic haemodialysis patients. Pharmacol Toxicol. 1990;66:83–6.

24. Lui SF, Wong KC, Li PKT, Lai KN. Once weekly versus twice weekly subcutaneous administration of recombinant human erythropoietin in haemodialysis patients. Am J Nephrol. 1992;12:55–60.

25. Besarab A, Nasca T, Ross R. Erythropoietin in patients prior to end-stage renal disease. Curr Opin Nephrol Hypertens. 1995;4:155–61.

26. Granneloras C, Branger B, Shaldon S, et al. Subcutaneous erythropoietin: a comparison of daily and thrice weekly administration. Contrib Nephrol. 1991;88: 144–51.
27. Sohmiya M, Kabika T, Kato Y. Therapeutic use of continued subcutaneous infusion of recombinant human erythropoietin in malnourished predialysis anemic patients with diabetic nephropathy. Eur J Endocrinol. 1998;139:367–70.
28. Besarab A, Bolton WK, Browne JK, Egrie JC, Nissenson AR, Okamato DM, Schwab SC, Goodkin DA. The effects of normal versus anemic hematocrit on hemodialysis patients with cardiac disease. N Eng J Med. 1998;339:584–90.
29. Ma JZ, Ebben J, Xia H, Collins AJ. Hematocrit level and associated mortality in hemodialysis patients. J Am Soc Nephrol. 1999;10:610–19.
30. Flaherty KK, Caro J, Erslev A, et al. Pharmacokinetics and erythropoietic response to human recombinant erythropoietin in healthy men. Clin Pharmacol Ther. 1990;47:557–64.
31. Eschbach JW, Abudulhadi MH, Browne JK, et al. Recombinant human erythro-poietin in anemic patients with end-stage renal disease: results of a phase III multi-center clinical trial. Ann Intern Med. 1989;111:992–1000.
32. Sabota JT. Recombinant human erythropoietin in patients with anemia due to end-stage renal disease. Contrib Nephrol. 1989; 76:166–78.
33. Walter J, Gal J, Taraba I. The beneficial effect of low initial dose and gradual increase of erythropoietin treatment in hemodialysis patients. Artif Organs. 1995;19:76–80.
34. Eschbach JW. Erythropoietin 1991 – An overview. Am J Kidney Dis. 1991;18 (supplement 4):3–9.
35. Caro J, Brown S, Miller OP, Murky T, Erslev AJ. Erythropoietin levels in uremic nephric and anephric patients. J Lab Clin Med. 1979;93:449–58.
36. Zaroulis CHG, Hoffman BJ, Kourides IA. Serum concentration of erythropoietin measured by radioimmunoassay in hematologic disorders and chronic renal failure. Am J Hematol. 1981;11:85–92.
37. Brockmoller J, Kochling J, Weber W, Looby M, Roots I, Neumayer H-H. The pharmacokinetics and pharmacodynamics or recombinant human erythropoie-tin in hemodialysis patients. Br J Clin Pharmacol. 1992;34:449–508.
38. Grannolleras C, Branger B, Beau MC, Deschodt G, Alsabadani B, Shaldon S. Experience with daily self-administered subcutaneous erythropoietin. Contrib Nephrol. 1989;76:143–8.
39. Macdougall IC, Gray SJ, Elston O, Breen C, Jenkins B, Browne J, Egrie J. Pharmacokinetics of novel erythropoiesis stimulating protein compared with epoetin alfa in dialysis patients. J Am Soc Nephrol. 1999;10:2392–5.

4. Is renal anemia management determined by science or reimbursement regulations?

Chaim Charytan

Regulatory and financial considerations have a long-standing, accepted and necessary role in the clinical decision-making process. Regulations define by whom, where and what services or procedures may be rendered. Since the inception of government funded health insurance, regulations also determine which and at what rate services will be compensated.

Financial considerations have an even older historical role in the decision-making process of health-care delivery. Can the patient afford the recommended therapy? Which of several therapeutic options is most economically suitable for the given individual? What is the potential socioeconomic impact of the illness and of the contemplated therapy on the patient and his family? Does the patient have insurance coverage? What services will it cover? In what setting, office, surgi-center or hospital are services covered? Does the patient have a drug plan that will pay for expensive medications such as erythrpoeitin (EPO) or parenteral iron?

Recently the proliferation of costly technological advances and the growing costs of medical care, in actual dollars and as a fraction of the national GNP, have given rise to initiatives aimed at making physicians even more sensitive to the economic aspects of medical care. Physicians are being asked to consider the global-societal economic consequences of clinical decisions made for individual patients. Training programs are encouraged to include a discussion of cost considerations in the training of residents in the clinical decision making process. There have even been suggestions that a system be developed for certifying physicians who practice "cost effective medicine."

It is also an accepted principle of medical practice to expect a payment rate that assures provider viability. This means a level of payment that covers all costs, including bad debt and unfunded care, and also allows a reasonable profit. In view of the above it would seem obvious that the answer to the question in the title of this presentation is that both science

Onyekachi Ifudu (ed.), Renal Anemia: Conflicts and Controversies. 29–35.
© 2002 Kluwer Academic Publishers.

and reimbursement regulations play a role in renal anemia management. What then is the significance and genesis of the question?

Perhaps a better understanding of the appropriateness of the question and the rationale for discussing this issue can be better understood by reviewing the fiscal impact of the End-Stage Renal Disease (ESRD) program on overall Medicare expenditures, the cost of anemia management in the dialysis population and the Health Care Finance Administration's (HCFA) response to these.

Current Medicare expenditures for ESRD care are in the range of 11 to 13 billion dollars [1]. This represents approximately six percent of the Medicare budget expended for only 0.8% of the Medicare population [2]. Furthermore, a progressive increase in expenditures is likely as a consequence of the projected 7 to 9% annual growth rate of the population requiring renal replacement therapy and continued technological advances, particularly the introduction of new and costly pharmaceuticals. The most obvious example is EPO. Payment for EPO contributes significantly to ESRD Medicare expenditures. In 1998, EPO accounted for 869 million, or 7% of total program expenditures [2].

A different perspective of the fiscal impact of payment for EPO on the ESRD program can be gleaned from the 2001 MedPac report to Congress [3]. That analysis demonstrates that the composite rate payment for dialysis services covers only 90%t of facility costs for these services. Facilities must rely on the profit margin for drug reimbursement, primarily EPO, to survive or to generate a small profit.

Analysis of payment for dialysis and ESRD outcomes in the United States, Europe and Japan reveals that the United States has the lowest reimbursement rates and the highest mortality rates of any industrialized nation [4,5]. A logical conclusion drawn from this data, by the Institute of Medicine [6] and by the MedPac [3], is that payment system for ESRD services is outdated, flawed and inadequate, and needs to be revamped and upgraded.

Conversely, HCFA's bureaucratic and paradoxical interpretation of the data is that EPO is overutilized for the purpose of generating facility profit and that nephrologists, even though most do not own dialysis facilities, are driven primarily by financial incentives in their EPO prescribing practices.

As a consequence of this attitude since the inception of the ESRD program, HCFA's coverage and payment policy has focused on cost containment, rather than encouragement and facilitation of quality outcomes [2,7,8]. This has been particularly true for regulations relating to EPO payment policy, which have changed four times since its introduction in 1989. Initially EPO was reimbursed at 40 dollars per administration for doses up to 9999 units and 70 dollars for doses larger than 10,000 units.

Not surprisingly, since few providers are able or willing to provide services at a loss, EPO doses were found to be inappropriately low and hematocrits inadequate. Consequently in 1990 Congress changed reimbursement to 11 dollars per thousand units. This was subsequently reduced to 10 dollars per thousand units through OBRA in 1994. The result was a marked improvement in hematocrit and hemoglobin levels, a dramatic decrease in transfusion requirements and an improved quality of life for maintenance hemodialysis patients [9].

While this represented a significant improvement in hematological status for the ESRD population, the mean hematocrit was only 31, well below the recommended standard of 33–36%. HCFA's Core Indicator Project [10], now the Clinical Performance Measures (CPM) project, and the NKF's DOQI guidelines [11] were launched in an effort to improve these and other outcomes in the ESRD dialysis population.

The renal community responded to these initiatives with a progressive increase in EPO utilization and hematocrit values [9,12]. As demonstrated in Figure 1, this trend was interrupted by the announcement of HCFA's intent to implement the hematocrit measurement audit (HMA) regulation.

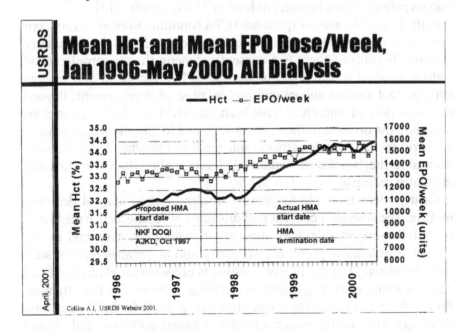

Figure 1.

This regulation precluded payment, without exception, for all EPO doses administered during a month in which the reported hematocrit was greater than 36% and the preceding three month rolling average hematocrit exceeded 36.5%. It was clearly understood, within the nephrology community, that the decline in mean hematocrits and EPO utilization was motivated by the need to avoid the very significant negative economic impact of this regulation.

This negative trend in ESRD anemia management continued during the the implementation of the HMA. It was reversed only after HCFA responded to an initiative spearheaded by the RPA on behalf of the renal community and once again modified the payment policy for EPO. The regulation, currently in force, does not penalize providers unless a three month rolling average hematocrit exceeds 37.5%. There is no regulatory limit to the level of any given month's hematocrit and some exceptions are permitted to the 37.5% ceiling. Announcement of this impending regulatory change resulted in an immediate increase in the average dose of EPO prescribed and a progressive increase in mean hematocrit in the dialysis population. In response to more liberal and biologically appropriate EPO payment policy, the CPM project, the DOQI guidelines and multiple educational and CQI initiatives by 1998, 65% of all in-center dialysis patients had a hematocrit level of 33% or greater [13].

In the face of the above experience HCFA continues to express a concern that physicians are prescribing excessive doses of EPO for pecuniary reasons. By contrast there is a consensus among the organizations and entities involved in the ESRD arena that EPO prescription and anemia management remain suboptimal and in need of improvement. Beyond that, a variety of initiatives have been launched to educate physicians regarding the needs to initiate EPO therapy and to improve hematocrits in the early, predialysis stages, of chronic renal insufficiency [14,15] and to determine the benefits of hematocrit levels higher than the currently mandated ceiling of 36.5% [16,17].

Clearly there is a role for fiscal considerations in clinical decision-making. The emerging concept and discipline of "cost-effective medicine" powerfully support this. It is also true that fiscal viability, and in our society, a reasonable profit, are necessary and acceptable goals of such considerations. Thus the proper question is not whether clinical or fiscal considerations drive physicians prescribing patterns for EPO therapy. Rather the correct question is what is the proper role for fiscal considerations and what is the proper interplay between economic and clinical considerations in the delivery of patient care?

The following questions should be asked in evaluating the appropriateness of the decision-making process. Is the primary goal an optimal clinical or economic outcome? Who is the primary beneficiary of the economic considerations: the patient, the provider, the payer or the global resource system, i.e., dollars available for overall care of the entire population? What are the goals of financial considerations: maintaining provider viability, preservation of resources, generating reasonable versus excessive profits? Do financial considerations drive the clinical decision-making process, or do they modify it and limit the options available for patient care?

A review of the history of EPO administration in the ESRD arena suggests that nephrologists have responded in a predictable and appropriate way to the regulatory changes, educational and CQI initiatives that have occurred since its introduction in 1989. Analysis of physicians' prescribing patterns in response to changes in EPO reimbursement policy, reflects an attempt to achieve optimal allowable hematocrit levels without jeopardizing provider fiscal viability. The majority of nephrologists, who do not own dialysis units, derive no financial benefit from EPO utilization. The data suggest that the nephrology community responded to educational and CQI initiatives, such as the Core Indicator Project (now the CPM), by increasing EPO utilization so as to maximize hemoglobin and hematocrit levels.

More recently in response to the DOQI guidelines and related educational initiatives there has been an increase in parenteral iron utilization, an increase in administration of EPO by the subcutaneous route, a further increase in the mean hematocrit level, and a decrease in EPO utilization in dialysis patients so treated. There is no data to suggest that, for the vast majority of physicians, inappropriate financial considerations were the driving force behind their prescribing patterns, nor that their intent was primarily to increase EPO utilization.

On the other hand, HCFA's EPO related regulations appear to have been driven primarily by fiscal considerations whose goal was stringent cost-containment [2,7,8]. It is difficult to otherwise explain some of the above-mentioned payment policy regulations and its expressed desire for an increase of subcutaneous EPO administration.

It is reasonable, though possibly overly idealistic, to expect that all participants in the health-care arena, including payers, have optimal clinical outcomes as the primary goal of their policy development process. Certainly this ought to be true for governmental regulatory and payment agencies. Their policies ought to be based on accepted standards of medical care, or where available evidence based medicine, as defined by the medical community. Quality care and optimal clinical outcomes should be the primary driving forces in this process. Fiscal concerns, limited economic resources and the need for cost-containment, are real and important issues, which ought to be discussed openly and not addressed through clinically inappropriate payment policies or regulations motivated by outliers. This approach would best serve all involved, payers, regulators, providers, patients and society.

REFERENCES

1. U.S. Renal Data System, USR DS 2000 Annual Data Report. National Institutes of Health, National Institute of Diabetes and Digestive and Kidney Diseases, Bethesda, MD, 753–838.
2. Eggers PW. A quarter century of Medicare expenditures for ESRD. Semin Nephrol. 2000;20:516–22.
3. MedPac. End-stage renal disease payment policies in traditional medicare. Report to the Congress: Medicare Payment Policy. March 2001:123–35.
4. Hull AR, Parker TF. Introduction and Summary: Proceedings from the Morbidity, Mortality and Prescription Dialysis Symposium, Dallas, TX. September 15–17, 1990. Am J Kidney Dis. 1990;15:3775–383.
5. Held PJ, Brunner F, Odaka M, et al. Five-year survival for ESRD patients in U.S., Europe and Japan, 1982–87. Am J Kidney Dis. 1990;15:451–7.
6. Rettig RA, Levinsky NG, eds. Kidney failure and the federal government: Committee for The Study of the Medicare End-Stage Renal Disease Program. Division of Health Care Services, Institute of Medicine, Washington D.C.: National Academy Press, 1991.
7. Hull AR. The legislative and regulatory process in the end-stage renal disease (ESRD) program, 1973 through 1997. Semin Nephrol. 1997;17:160–9.
8. Farley DO. Financing of end-stage renal disease care: past, present, and future. Adv Renal Replacement Ther. 1994;1:24–31.
9. Collins AJ, Ma JZ, Xia A, et al. Trends in anemia treatment with erythrpoeitin usage and patient outcomes. Am J Kidney Dis. 1998;32:S133–41.
10. 1995 Annual Reports: ESRD Core Indicators Project. Department of Health And Human Services, Health Care Financing Administration, and Health Standards Quality Bureau, January, 1996.
11. National Kidney Foundation-Dialysis Outcomes Quality Initiative. NKF-DOQI clinical practice guidelines for the treatment of anemia of chronic renal failure. Am J Kidney Dis. 1997;30(4 supplement 3):S192–240.
12. Collins AJ, Agodoa LYC, Eggers PW. USRDS assessment of clinical care of dialysis patients, 2001. <http://www.usrds.org/pres/NKF/NKFDOQI>.
13. Health Care Financing Administration 1999 Annual Report, End-stage Renal Disease Clinical Performance Measures Project, Baltimore, MD. Department Of Health And Human Services, Health Care Financing Administration, Office of Clinical Standards and Quality, 1999.
14. Obrador GT, Arora P, Kausz AT, Pereira BJ. Pre-end-stage renal disease care in the United States: a state of disrepair. J Am Soc Nephrol. 1998;9(12 supplement): S44–54.

15. Nissenson AR, Collins AJ, Hurley J, et al. Opportunities for improving the care of patients with chronic renal insufficiency: current practice patterns. J Am Soc Nephrol. 2001;12:1713–20.
16. Besarab A, Aslam MA. Should the hematocrit (hemoglobin) been normalized in pre-ESRD or dialysis patients? Yes! Blood Purif. 2001;19:168–74.
17. Foley RN, Parfrey PS, Morgan J, et al. Effect of hemoglobin levels in hemodialysis patients with asymptomatic cardiomyopathy. Kidney Int. 2000;58:1325–35.

5. When does anemia impact the heart in chronic kidney disease?

Adeera Levin

It is well documented that patients with kidney disease have a high burden of cardiovascular illness. CVD can be simplistically categorized into disorders of perfusion and disorders of pump function [1]. Both can co-exist, and one can exacerbate the other. Importantly, disorders of perfusion may well be due to atherosclerotic processes, while disorders of pump function can be due to ischemic damage (the result of perfusion disorders), but are also related to abnormalities of left ventricular geometry and growth, which may be propagated by specific components present in uremic milieu. Using a similar dichotomous approach, risk factors for cardiovascular disease (CVD) in patients with kidney disease can be categorized into both "traditional" and "uremia-related", which would correspond to those factors impacting vasculature (perfusion) and those impacting pump function.

Traditional risk factors include smoking, dyslipidemia, hypertension, diabetes, and positive family history, while risk factors that are character-istic of uremia include anemia, hyperparathyroidism, and decline in kidney function. Both traditional and uremia related risk factors may be operational in one individual, or may interact to adversely impact on outcome. Of interest is that therapeutic strategies are available for both categories of risk factors.

The role of anemia has received substantial attention in the dialysis population. Anemia in particular has been correlated with the presence of left ventricular hypertrophy (LVH), congestive heart failure (CHF) (at both dialysis initiation and over the first year of dialysis), and symptoms of angina and heart failure [2]. There is increasing evidence that anemia is important in patients with chronic kidney disease, prior to dialysis, and this article attempts to focuses on advances in the understanding of the complex relationship of anemia, CVD, and CKD.

Onyekachi Ifudu (ed.), Renal Anemia: Conflicts and Controversies, 37–47.
© *2002 Kluwer Academic Publishers.*

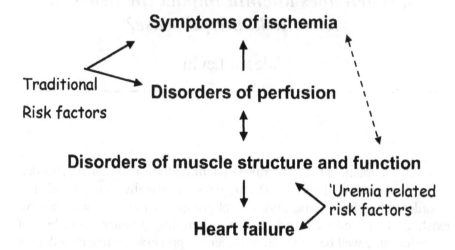

Cardiovascular disease

Figure 1. Demonstrates a schematic representation of cardiac disease, dichotomously characterized as disorders of perfusion and of pump function. Traditional and uremic risk factors are shown as preferentially affecting one or the other. See text for details. Adapted from Parfrey [1], and personal communication.

Defining anemia

Firstly, it is essential to define anemia. According to the World Health Organization, (WHO) anemia is defined in physiological terms, according to gender and menstrual status. Thus, in men, levels of Hgb <13.5 gm/dl and in post menopausal or non menstruating women, Hgb levels of <12.5 gm/dl are considered evidence of anemia. Note however, in most populations of kidney disease, that anemia is referred to as that Hgb less than target levels of 12 gm/dl, and is traditionally not treated until levels of 10 g/dl are achieved. Much of this is determined or inadvertently regulated by reimbursement practices: interestingly, practices are similar across different countries [3,4].

Traditionally in patients with kidney disease, the term "renal anemia" has been used to both identify a fall in hemoglobin, attributable to kidney disease itself. Concomitantly, the term has also been used to identify a threshold of hemoglobin below patients require treatment. This leads to the subliminal acceptance of non physiological targets in this group of patients, and may account for many of current practice patterns, and perhaps to ongoing links between hemoglobin levels and the poor outcomes of these patients. In reviewing the impact of anemia in patients with CKD, prior to dialysis, it is important to use physiologic definitions, so as to gain the best understanding of the impact of a fall in hemoglobin.

CVD IN CKD

Spectrum of disease

Cardiovascular mortality rates among patients with end-stage renal disease (ESRD) are significantly higher than are those among the general population, even when adjustments are made for age, gender, and diabetic status. Data for the dialysis and transplant populations are well described in numerous publications [5,6]. Interestingly, cardiovascular mortality rates in transplant recipients, a model of gradual CKD, are noted to be between those rates described for the general population and those for dialysis patients. Note that these patients have been exposed to CKD "milieu" prior to receiving a transplant, and thus have an exposure to those risk factors associated with uremia.

In contrast to our understanding of CVD in dialysis and transplant populations, the understanding in CKD patients is limited. This is due to numerous factors, including issues of survivor bias, incomplete registration or follow up of patients not on dialysis, or late referral/non referral to nephrologists.

However, in recent publications, a consistent pattern is demonstrated. The prevalence of CVD, defined as CHF, angina, history of MI, TIA or PVD, is approximately 38–40% in patients with established chronic kidney disease seen by nephrologists [1,7]. In cardiac interventional registries and CCU admission data bases, patients with impaired kidney function do less well (increased morbidity and mortality relative to those with normal kidney function) [8–10]. Accumulating data suggests that the rates exceed those seen in the general population [11]. Left ventricular enlargement is common, and in CKD, with an inverse relationship between the prevalence of LVH and kidney function [12–14] has been described.

Anemia and cardiovascular disease

The association of anemia with CVD has been noted in dialysis patients by numerous investigators [5,11,12,15,16]. It is clear that there is excessive CV morbidity in association with anemia in dialysis populations. In

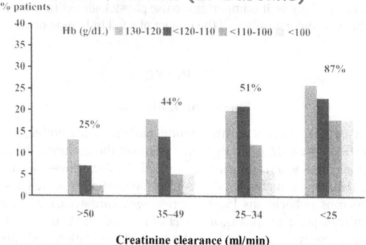

Prevalence of 'anemia' by degree of renal function (at baseline)

Creatinine clearance (ml/min)

p<0.05 between all categories

Levin et al. *AJKD*, 1999

Figure 2. This demonstrates the prevalence of hemoglobin values at level of kidney function, estimated by creatinine clearance, in a cohort of patients prior to dialysis. Upper limit of hemoglobin selected is 13, which is below the level of hemoglobin which defines anemia according to World Health Organization. The prevalence of anemia increases at each lower level of kidney function, with the prevalence reaching 87% in the lowest group. This data is adapted from the data by Levin et al. [14].

addition, hemoglobin levels have been shown to be associated with cardiac hospitalizations in patients prior to dialysis [13,17], and to predict morbidity and mortality in HD patients [18].

Most consistently, anemia is associated with left ventricular hypertrophy, with congestive heart failure and with a lesser extent to ischemic heart disease. The strong associations between level of hemoglobin and LVH or heart failure is described in dialysis patients and in those prior to dialysis [5,11–13,15,16]. Recent publications by Rigatto et al. extend these observations of a consistent relationship of hemoglobin and heart disease/function in transplanted patients. In a cohort of patients followed post transplant, hemoglobin level predicted the advent of de novo CHF events [6,19].

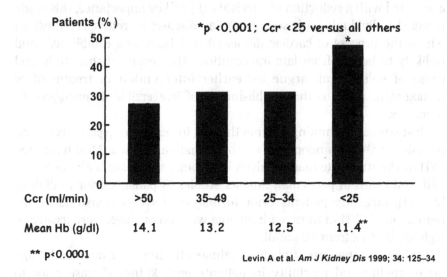

Figure 3. This figure demonstrates the increasing prevalence of LVH in patients prior to dialysis, as a function of category of creatinine clearance, mean hemoglobin values are displayed under each level of kidney function. Note the ranges of hemoglobin are within current dialysis target ranges. This is data adapted from Levin et al. [14].

Importantly, there is less clear association of hemoglobin and ischemic heart disease events (angina and MI) than there is with heart failure. This is underscores the need to conceptualize pump function and perfusion disorders separately. The relationship to ischemic events may be confounded by survival bias in cohort studies, or over ridden by other factors contributing to atherosclerosis *per se*. Thus, anemia my impact on CV disease in two ways: firstly by its indirect effect on cardiac structure, through the induction of LVH, and secondly indirectly by limiting oxygen delivery in the presence of atherosclerotic or arteriosclerotic lesions.

Treatment trials

Unlike interventional trials in cardiology, the results of interventional studies in kidney patients have been limited by sample size, use of surrogate measures for CVD, duration or targets of therapy, or selection of specific populations. In hemodialysis patients, anemia therapy has been demonstrated to reduce LV dilatation in asymptomatic HD patients with LVH [20]. In the oft quoted Normalization of Hemoglobin study published in NEJM, normalization of hemoglobin did not improve, and in fact, was associated with a reduction in survival [21]. Of key importance, this study targeted individuals with severe cardiac disease: in retrospect those in whom the process of cardiac disease(s) had been well established, and unlikely to benefit from late intervention. The results of this study and those of Foley et al. argue for earlier intervention in treatment of hemoglobin, prior to the establishment of irreversible damage/growth processes.

Most studies examining anemia therapy in nephrology patients not on dialysis are a) non-randomized, and b) of small sample size. Most have used LVH as the surrogate marker, given its strong association with outcomes, CHF and death in particular. Smaller studies in patients prior to dialysis [22–24], targeting patients prior to dialysis, have demonstrated some regression of LVH in those with anemia who, on average, were treated to Hgb levels of 12 from 10 gm/dl.

To date, no long-term study has evaluated the impact of anemia therapy on morbidity and mortality in patients with kidney disease prior to dialysis. However, several studies are currently in progress in the US, Canada and internationally, in Europe, and Australia.

Why should it be that anemia impacts CVD so dramatically and consistently in patients with kidney disease?

The relationship between lower hemoglobin levels and CVD outcomes (LVH and CHF or hospitalizations for cardiac problems) is consistently demonstrated in a number of populations: prior to dialysis, on dialysis and post transplant. The impact of level of hemoglobin has been shown to be independent of kidney function, in non dialysis patients, and thus not simply a marker for poor kidney function. Hemoglobin is well recognized as essential for oxygen delivery to tissues and vital organs, thus reduction in oxygen delivery stimulates a variety of adaptive responses that ultimately culminate in processes related to CVD expression.

Hypoxia will necessarily stimulate compensatory mechanisms at both whole organ and cellular levels. Increase in cardiac output and heart rate and contractility is achieved through vasodilatation and increase in sympathetic activity. These ultimately lead to volume included LV dilatation (eccentric LVH). The increase in oxygen extraction facilitated by the increase in 2,3 DPG and cellular adaptation can compensate for approximately 1-2 g/dl changes in Hgb, but after that, the increases in sympathetic system activation, mediated by cytokines and growth factors become prominent.

Superimposed on this set of anemia related events, are those related to kidney disease itself: increases in plasma volume and hypertension, mediated in part by the renal angiotensin system, lead to pressure induced (concentric) LVH. As well, other factors (such as hyperparathyroidism, abnormalities of calcium and phosphate) may contribute to the process of LV growth and the change in myofibril constitution or orientation. Usually these processes of concentric and eccentric LVH occur concomitantly and continuously throughout the duration of kidney disease [25–28].

The consequences of LVH are subsequently exacerbated by lower hemoglobin, especially in the presence of established CAD (both micro and macro-vascular disease) [31]. The increase in number of myocardial ischemia events, has been shown to increase 3–6 fold [10], as has the incidence of heart failure. While the issues of factors affecting cardiac structure/function versus those affecting perfusion (atherosclerosis and arteriosclerosis) may well be separate, they are undoubtedly related in patients with kidney disease [1].

Anemia defined physiologically and CVD: rationale for conclusions and new directions

Historically, most studies have defined anemia *a priori* using threshold values of hemoglobin < 10 g/dL or hematocrit < 28%. More recently it has been determined that even at higher absolute levels of hemoglobin, a relative decrease from baseline can be associated with left ventricular growth, thus providing strong evidence that earlier attention to changes in hemoglobin values in CKD patients is important [22,30]. Further corroboration of this concept can be obtained from recent studies such as that by Hayashi's group, in which regression of LVH was achieved after hemoglobin levels were corrected to values above those currently recommended for dialysis populations [22]. The relative risk for an increase in left ventricular mass has been reproducibly estimated to be in the range of 1.32 to 1.60 for each gram of hemoglobin decrease [16], indicating again the powerful association of anemia on patient outcomes.

In an intriguing recent observation by Silverberg and colleagues [31], 26 patients with a history of refractory class IV CHF who were identified as being "relatively" anemic (mean entry hemoglobin of 10.16 ± 0.95 g/dl) were treated with erythropoietin and iron. Treatment of the relative anemia in this fashion achieved a mean hemoglobin of 12.10 ± 1.21 g/dl and resulted in major reductions in symptoms, hospital visits, and inpatient admissions relative to baseline. Of note, the 26 patients who were treated prospectively had a mean entry serum creatinine value of 2.59 ± 0.77 mg/dl, signifying a moderate to severe degree of kidney disease.

Although the sample size was small and the trial was not randomized or controlled, it emphasizes the importance of recognizing and aggressively managing anemia in patients with CKD and CVD. Note is made that the level of 12 gm/dl was the mean Hgb value achieved, which is well above current usual initiation levels in dialysis populations. At this level, substantial disease burden already exists.

Treatment of anemia: strategies and outcomes

The regression of LVH is an achievable goal, as demonstrated by several small studies cited above [22–24,31]. These studies all imply that earlier therapy of anemia, in asymptomatic phases of heart disease and/or prior to the development of irreversible myocardial structural changes, may be extremely beneficial in CKD patients. The definitive prospective studies are currently under way to examine these issues more rigorously than has been done previously.

Important for clinicians to remember, is that the correction of anemia in renal patients does reverse a number of the associated hemodynamic alterations, including the characteristic changes in peripheral vascular resistance, stroke volume, and cardiac output. It is therefore logical that such treatment, provided early enough, would reduce the propensity to left ventricular enlargement. In fact, reductions as dramatic as 10% to 30% have been documented using treatment strategies that include iron supplementation, erythropoietin, and, in selected cases, red blood cell transfusions [24,31]. Treatment of anemia is also associated with other benefits including improved quality of life, cognitive function, and exercise tolerance.

Other CVD risk factors

In addition to anemia, other factors that contribute to the CVD burden of patients with CKD include hypertension and numerous coexisting metabolic aberrations (e.g., dyslipidemia, diabetes mellitus, hyperparathyroidism). The focus of this paper is to underscore the important and perhaps unique role of anemia in this population. The relative impact of anemia in conjunction, with or without these other factors, is not yet fully understood.

The importance of blood pressure control, achieving target BP levels below 130/80 mmHg, is important in delaying the progression of kidney disease but is also essential in reducing the endothelial damage, subsequent shear stresses on vessels, and acceleration of atherosclerotic lesions known to occur in the uremic milieu. A number of agents including angiotensin-converting enzyme inhibitors, angiotensin receptor blockers, calcium channel blockers, and β-blockers all have been shown to be beneficial in high-risk patient groups [10]. The relationship of these drugs to propagation or acceleration of fall in hemoglobin is still under investigation.

Given that there is accumulating data for primary and secondary prevention in improving CVD outcomes in general populations, it is reasonable to view patients with CKD as being at high risk for these events, and thus warranting aggressive risk factor reduction strategies.

SUMMARY

The spectrum of CVD in patients with CKD includes LVH, left ventricular dilatation, ischemic heart disease, and peripheral vascular disease. Both traditional and uremia-specific risk factors contribute to the prevalence of these disorders in patients with kidney disease. Anemia, defined in physiological terms, as hemoglobin levels below 13.5 g/L and 12.5 g/L, is clearly associated with CVD. Evidence is accumulating that the processes contributing to CVD commence early in kidney disease. Modifiable risk factors include hypertension, anemia, hyperparathyroidism, and dyslipidemia, and all are amenable to therapy. Earlier intervention, appropriate definition, and thus treatment of factors such as anemia, may offer the best opportunity to reduce the burden of illness in patients with kidney disease. It is of critical importance that nephrologists help to identify patients with kidney disease, delineate the extent and impact of the known risk factors for CVD, and participate in appropriately powered randomized control trials. It is through the application of the scientific method, and long-term interventional studies, that the community will be able to determine costs, benefits, and risks of therapeutic strategies, alone and in combination.

REFERENCES

1. Parfrey P. Is renal insufficiency an atherogenic state? Reflections on prevalence, incidence and risk. Am J Kidney Dis. 2001;37:154–7.

2.   Foley RN, Parfrey PS, Harnett JD, et al. Clinical and echocardiographic disease in patients starting end-stage renal disease therapy. Kidney Int. 1995;47:186–92.
3.   European Survey on Anemia Management (ESAM) Nephrol Dial Transplantation. 2000;15(supplement 4).
4.   USRDS: Annual Data Report V. Patient mortality and survival. Am J Kidney Dis. 1998;32(supplement 1): S69–S80. United States Renal Data System. USRDS 1998 Annual Report. Bethesda, MD: National Institutes of Health, National Institute of Diabetes and Digestive and Kidney Diseases; 1998.
5.   Parfrey PS, Foley RN, Harnett JD, Kent GM, Murray DC, Barre PE. Outcome and risk factors for left ventricular disorders in chronic uremia. Nephrol Dial Transplantation. 1996;11:1277—85.
6.   Rigatto C, Foley R, Kent G, et al. Long term changes in left ventricular hypertrophy following renal transplantation. Transplantation. 2000;70:570–5.
7.   Levin A , Djurdjev O, Barrett B, Burgess E, et al. Cardiovascular disease in patients with chronic kidney disease: getting to the heart of the matter. Am J Kidney Dis. 2001;38:1398–407
8.   Hemmelgarn BC, Ghali WAS, Quan HB, et al. for the APPROACH investigators. Poor long term survival after coronary angiogram in patients with renal insufficiency. Am J Kidney Dis. 2001;37:64–72.
9.   Beattie JN, Soman SS, Sandberg KR, Yee J, Borzak S, McCullough PA. Determinants of mortality after myocardial infarction in patients with advanced renal dysfunction. Am J Kidney Dis. 2001;37:1191–200.
10.   Mann J, Gertstein, HC, Pogue J, Baosch, Yusef, S for the Hope Investigators. Renal insufficiency as a predictor cardiovascular outcomes and the impact of ramipril: The Hope Randomized Trial. Ann Intern Med. 2001;134(8):629–36.
11.   Foley RN, Parfrey PS. Cardiovascular disease and mortality in ESRD. J Nephrol. 1998;11:239–45.
12.   Greaves SC, Gamble GD, Collins JF, Whalley GA, Sharpe DN. Determinants of left ventricular hypertrophy and systolic dysfunction in chronic renal failure. Am J Kidney Dis. 1994;24:768–76.
13.   Levin A, Singer J, Thompson CR, Ross H, Lewis M. Prevalent left ventricular hypertrophy in the predialysis population: identifying opportunities for intervention. Am J Kidney Dis. 1996;27:347–54.
14.   Levin A, Thompson C, Either J, Carlisle E, Tobe S, Mendelssohn D, Burgess E, Jindal K, Barrett B, Singer J, Djurdjev O. Left ventricular mass index increase in early renal disease: Impact of decline in hemoglobin. Am J Kidney Dis. 1999;34:125–34.
15.   Parfrey PS, Harnett JD, Foley RN. Heart failure and ischemic heart disease in chronic uremia. Curr Opin Nephrol Hypertens. 1995;4:105–10.
16.   Harnett JD, Kent GM, Foley RN, Parfrey PS. Cardiac function and hematocrit level. Am J Kidney Dis. 1995;25:S3–S7.
17.   Holland DC, Lam M. Predictors of hospitalization and death among pre-dialysis patients: a retrospective cohort study. Nephrol Dial Transplantation. 2000;15:650–8.
18.   Collins AJ, Ma JZ, Xia A, Ebben J. Trends in anemia treatment with erythropoietin usage and patient outcomes. Am J Kidney Dis. 1998;32:S133–S141.
19.   Rigatto C. Cardiac disease in renal transplant recipients. Masters theses, Memorial University Department of Epidemiology, June 2001.
20.   Foley RN, Parfrey PS , Morgan J, Barre P, Campbell P, Cartier P, et al. Effect of hemoglobin levels in hemodialysis patients with asymptomatic cardiomyopathy. Kidney Int. 2000;58:1325–35.
21.   Besarab A, Bolton W, Browne J, Egrie J, Nissenson A, Okamoto D, Schwab S, Goodkin D. The effects of normal as compared with low hematocrit values in

patients with cardiac disease receiving hemodialysis and epoetin. N Engl J Med. 1998;339:584–90.

22. Hayashi T, Suzuki A, Shoji T, Togawa M, Okada N, Tsubakihara Y, Imai E, Hori M. Cardiovascular effect of normalizing the hematocrit level during erythropoietin therapy in predialysis patients with chronic renal failure. Am J Kidney Dis. 2000; 35:250–6.

23. Kuriyama S, Tomonari H, Yoshida H, Hashimoto T, Kawaguchi Y, Sakai O. Reversal of anemia by erythropoietin therapy retards progression of chronic renal failure, especially in nondiabetic patients. Nephron. 1997;77:176–85.

24. Portoles J, Torralbo A, Martin P, Rodrigo J, Herrero J, Barrientos A. Cardiovascular effects of recombinant human erythropoietin in pre-dialysis patients. Am J Kidney Dis. 1997;29:541–8.

25. Hunter JJ, Chien KR. Signalling pathways for cardiac hypertrophy and failure. N Engl J Med. 1999;341:1276–83.

26. Amann K, Kronenberg G, Gehlen F, et al. Cardiac remodelling in experimental renal failure–an immunohistochemical study. Nephrol Dial Transplantation. 1998;13:1958–66.

27. London GM, Fabiani F, Marchais SJ, et al. Uremic cardiomyopathy: an inadequate left ventricular hypertrophy. Kidney Int. 1987;31:973–80.

28. Middleton, Rachel J, Parfrey P, Foley R. Left ventricular hypertrophy in the renal patient. J Am Soc Nephrol. 2001;12:1079–84.

29. Eckardt KU. Cardiovascular consequences of renal anaemia and erythropoietin therapy. Nephrol Dial Transplantation. 1999;14:1317–23.

30. Murphy SW, Foley RN, Barrett BJ, et al. Comparative hospitalization of hemodialysis and peritoneal dialysis patients in canada. Kidney Int. 2000;57: 2557–63.

31. Silverberg D, Wexler D, Blum M, Keren G, Sheps D, Laibovitch E, Brosh D, Laniado S, Schwartz D, Yachnin T, Shapira I, Gavish D, Baruch R, Koifman B, Kaplan C, Steinbruch S, Iaina A. The use of subcutaneous erythropoietin and intravenous iron for the treatment of the anemia of severe, resistant congestive heart failure improves cardiac and renal function and functional cardiac class, and markedly reduces hospitalizations. J Am Coll Cardiol. 2000;35:1737–44.

6. Improvements in anemia management with darbepoetin alfa, a new erythropoiesis stimulating protein

Jill S. Lindberg

INTRODUCTION

There is a high prevalence of chronic kidney disease (CKD) and associated anemia in the United States (US). The Third National Health and Nutrition Examination Survey of 18,723 participants estimated that there are as many as 6.2 million people in the US with a serum creatinine (SCr) level of 1.5 mg/dl or above [1].

CKD is a significant public health problem. It is associated with diabetes and hypertension, and results in many complications including cardio-vascular disease, anemia, and hyperalbuminemia. Early identification of patients with CKD and prompt treatment is essential to prevent these complications and to slow the progression to end-stage renal disease (ESRD)[2]. This would not only improve patient outcomes, but would also constrain the growth in costs of patients entering dialysis and transplant programs.

Anemia is one of the most characteristic findings of CKD, and develops as renal function falls below 50% of normal [2]. Studies indicate that approximately 40% of CKD patients (SCr ≥ 2.0 mg/dl for males and ≥ 1.5 mg/dl for females) are anemic (hematocrit 30%) [3], with the prevalence of anemia directly correlated with the severity of renal insufficiency. One analysis of anemic patients beginning dialysis in the US found that 67% had a hematocrit of less than 30% and 51% had a hematocrit of less than 28% [4].

Anemia may present with various symptoms, including fatigue, weakness, angina, and shortness of breath. When untreated, anemia causes or contributes to insomnia, depression, cognitive dysfunction, decreased libido, and left ventricular hypertrophy [5,6]. CKD patients with anemia

Onyekachi Ifudu (ed.), Renal Anemia: Conflicts and Controversies, 49–64.

have an impaired quality of life, a greater need for red blood cell transfusions, increased hospitalizations, and increased risk of death [5,7].

Anemia in CKD is primarily caused by a deficiency in endogenous erythropoietin (EPO) [8]. EPO is produced by the kidneys in response to a fall in oxygen delivery to the renal parenchyma. Diseases destroying the tubulo-interstitial cells of the kidney, which are responsible for EPO production, are major causes of renal anemia. In addition to the relative lack of EPO, increased red blood cell destruction and loss must be considered as possible causes contributing to renal anemia [9].

Endogenous EPO deficiency can be corrected by the administration of recombinant human erythropoietin (rHuEPO, epoetin alfa), and by the new erythropoiesis stimulating protein, darbepoetin alfa (Aranesp™, Amgen Inc., Thousand Oaks, CA) [10–12]. The management of anemia with rHuEPO (epoetin alfa) and darbepoetin alfa is reviewed in this chapter.

Current management of anemia with rHuEPO

rHuEPO was developed following the breakthrough in the isolation and cloning of the EPO gene by Lin and colleagues [13]. Since its marketing approval by the Food and Drug Administration (FDA) in 1989, rHuEPO has transformed the management of anemia in patients with CKD [14,15]. Therapy with rHuEPO has improved the clinical outcomes and quality of life for patients with CKD including those on and not on dialysis [16–18]. Prior to the introduction of rHuEPO, management of anemia patients was poor, and treatment with blood transfusions and androgenic steroids was required, often with significant adverse effects and complications [19].

Patients can receive rHuEPO intravenously (IV), subcutaneously (SC), or intraperitoneally (IP). The half-life of IV rHuEPO is 4–9 hours and greater than 24 hours when given SC [20]. The time to peak concentration after SC administration is usually more than 10 hours, while the range in bioavailability is large and ranges from 16% to 50% [21].

The initial recommended IV dose of rHuEPO in adults is 50–100 U/kg administered three times per week [22]. When given SC to patients with ESRD, rHuEPO is generally initiated at a dose of 80–120 U/kg and given as two or three doses per week [23]. The dose that is initially selected should, as outlined in the National Kidney Foundation (NKF) Kidney Disease Outcomes Quality Initiative (K/DOQI™) guidelines, achieve a target hemoglobin level of 11–12 g/dl or hematocrit of 33–36% within a period of 2–4 months [24].

rHuEPO is generally safe and well tolerated. There is an association with the use of rHuEPO and the development or worsening of pre-existing hypertension within weeks or months of its initiation in approximately 25% of treated patients [25,26]. Other reported adverse effects include vascular access thrombosis [27] and hyperkalemia [11,27,28], but it has not been demonstrated convincingly that these are adverse effects related to rHuEPO.

The current dosing recommendation for rHuEPO to be administered three times weekly places a limitation on its use in patients who do not attend clinics on such a frequent basis [22,29]. Frequent administration can place a burden on patients and healthcare staff. Thus, a longer acting erythropoietic agent, which can be administered less frequently, could potentially alleviate some of these difficulties. Darbepoetin alfa, a new erythropoiesis stimulating protein, is a long-acting drug and can be administered less frequently than rHuEPO [12]. The ease of use of this drug simplifies anemia management in patients with CKD, and could help alleviate the under-treatment of anemia. This is especially important in patients with early CKD who do not attend renal clinics on a frequent basis.

The development of darbepoetin alfa

Darbepoetin alfa is the first of a new generation of erythropoietic proteins. It is biochemically distinct from rHuEPO but stimulates erythropoiesis by the same mechanism as natural and recombinant EPO. Darbepoetin alfa binds to the EPO receptor on the surface of red blood cell precursors in the bone marrow and sets off an intracellular signaling mechanism involving receptor tyrosine phosphorylation [30]. This stimulates the proliferation and differentiation of red blood cell precursors and prolongs their survival by inhibiting apoptosis in the same way as EPO. The concentration of hemoglobin in the blood is increased, thus, treating the anemia.

The discovery of darbepoetin alfa arose from research into the factors and structural features that control the *in vivo* activity of EPO. Studies of EPO demonstrated a direct relationship between the sialylated carbohydrate content and its half-life and *in vivo* biological activity [30,31].

The amino acid sequence of rHuEPO was re-engineered to introduce new N-linked carbohydrate recognition sequences, Asn-Xxx-Thr/Ser [32]. The newly created proteins were tested for the presence of glycosylation at the new sites as well as their ability to stimulate the EPO receptor. Combination of two successfully glycosylated four-chain proteins into one molecule led to the formation of darbepoetin alfa. Darbepoetin alfa contains five N-linked carbohydrate chains, whereas rHuEPO contains three (Figure 1). This gives darbepoetin alfa an increased molecular weight and greater negative charge [30].

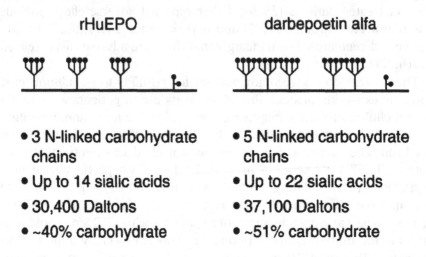

Figure 1. Comparison of the structure and biochemical properties of rHuEPO and darbepoetin alfa [12].

Experimentation into the pharmacokinetics and biological activity of darbepoetin alfa showed that it had a longer half-life than rHuEPO in animals, and that there was a dose-dependent increase in hemoglobin levels in normal mice injected with darbepoetin alfa by the IV, IP, and SC routes [30].

Overall, there was a 3.6-fold increase in the *in vivo* efficacy of darbepoetin alfa compared with rHuEPO when each molecule was administered three times per week. However, when each molecule was administered once-weekly, darbepoetin alfa was found to be 13- to 14-fold more effective at raising hematocrit levels. Darbepoetin alfa administered once-weekly was as effective as the same weekly dose of rHuEPO administered as three divided doses (Figure 2) [30].

A comparison of the pharmacokinetics of darbepoetin alfa with rHuEPO

Pharmacokinetic studies in humans have confirmed that darbepoetin alfa has a longer serum half-life than rHuEPO and can thus be administered less frequently. In a double-blind, randomized, cross-over study of

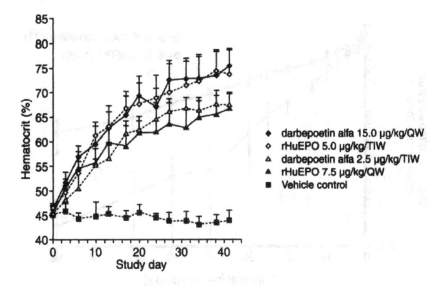

Figure 2. Comparative efficacy of darbepoetin alfa administered once-weekly (QW) and rHuEPO administered three times per week (TIW) in CD-1 mice [30].

peritoneal dialysis patients, the single-dose pharmacokinetics of rHuEPO (100 U/kg) and darbepoetin alfa (an equimolar dose) were compared following IV administration (Figure 3) [33]. In all patients, darbepoetin alfa had a longer terminal half-life than rHuEPO.

As summarized in Table 1, the mean terminal half-life for darbepoetin alfa following IV injection was 25.3 hours, approximately three times longer than that determined for rHuEPO (8.5 hours). After SC administration, the mean terminal elimination half-life for darbepoetin alfa was 48.8 hours, which was twice as long as that for IV darbepoetin alfa. Darbepoetin alfa had a significantly greater area under the serum concentrationtime curve (AUC), and clearance was lower compared with similar doses of rHuEPO. The volume of distribution for darbepoetin alfa was similar to that of rHuEPO (52.4 ml/kg vs. 48.7 ml/kg). The mean bioavailability of darbepoetin alfa was 36.9% [33], which was similar to that reported for SC rHuEPO.

The pharmacokinetics of darbepoetin alfa following chronic IV [34] and SC [35] administration confirmed that the elimination half-life of darbepoetin alfa, administered IV three times per week or once-weekly, was again approximately three times longer compared with IV rHuEPO given three times weekly. The pharmacokinetics of chronic IV therapy were both

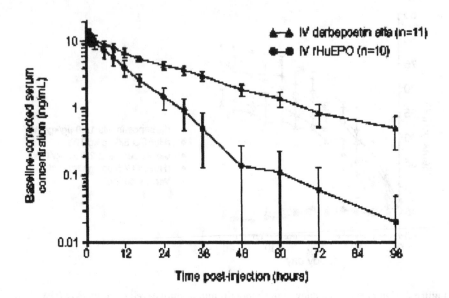

Figure 3. Comparative pharmacokinetics of darbepoetin alfa and epoetin alfa in anemic dialysis patients. Results are expressed as the mean (±SD). Reproduced with the permission of Lippincott Williams and Wilkins [33].

Table 1. Comparison of the mean pharmacokinetic pararmeters of intravenous rHuEPO with intravenous darbepoetin alfa [33]

Parameter	IV rHuEPO (n = 10)	IV darbepoetin alfa (n = 11)
$t_{\frac{1}{2}z}$ (h) 8.5	25.3	
AUC (mg/h/L)*	131.9	291.0
CL (ml/h/kg)	4.0	1.6
V_d (ml/kg)	48.7	52.4

$t_{\frac{1}{2}z}$, terminal phase elimination half-life; T_{max}, time to maximum serum concentration; AUC, area under serum concentrationtime curve; CL, clearance; V_d, volume of distribution at steady state

dose- and time-linear and there was no evidence of accumulation over 48 weeks of treatment [34].

The pharmacokinetics of IV and SC darbepoetin alfa in pediatric patients with CKD were found to be similar to those in adults [36]. However, darbepoetin alfa may be absorbed more rapidly in pediatric patients (mean T_{max}: 36.2 hours in children versus 54.1 hours in adults), an effect that has also been observed with rHuEPO [37].

These pharmacokinetic studies confirm that darbepoetin alfa has an approximately two- to three-fold longer half-life compared with rHuEPO, enabling it to be administered less frequently than traditional anemia therapy.

An evaluation of the clinical trial data for darbepoetin alfa in CKD patients with anemia

The clinical development program for darbepoetin alfa in patients with CKD has involved over 2000 patients from 15 studies conducted across North America, Europe, Australia, and South America. These studies have examined the efficacy and safety of darbepoetin alfa in managing anemia in patients with early CKD and those on dialysis.

Correction of anemia in rHuEPO-naive CKD patients not on dialysis

Clinical studies have shown that darbepoetin alfa is effective at correcting anemia in patients with CKD at a reduced dosing frequency compared with rHuEPO [38,39]. In one study, patients with early CKD who had a creatinine clearance less than 30 ml/min, were not yet on dialysis, and had hemoglobin levels less than 11 g/dL were randomized to receive darbepoetin alfa 0.45 µg/kg SC once-weekly (n = 129), or rHuEPO, 50 U/kg SC twice-weekly (n = 37). The rHuEPO dose was approximately 10% higher than the total weekly dose of darbepoetin alfa.

A similar proportion of patients were found to have achieved a hemoglobin response (hemoglobin increase [3]1 g/dL from baseline and a hemoglobin concentration [3]11 g/dL) in the two treatment groups (93% darbepoetin alfa, 92% rHuEPO). The mean rise in hemoglobin after 4 weeks of treatment was also similar (1.38 g/dL darbepoetin alfa, 1.40 g/dl rHuEPO). The median time to achieve a hemoglobin response was 7 weeks in both groups (Figure 4). At the time of the peak hemoglobin response, the median weekly dose was 0.46 µg/kg for darbepoetin alfa and 100 U/kg for rHuEPO [38]. After correction of anemia, target hemoglobin concentrations were maintained with a median darbepoetin alfa dose of 0.34 µg/kg [38,40]. The study showed that darbepoetin alfa administered once-weekly by the SC route at a starting dose of 0.45 µg/kg is well tolerated and as effective as rHuEPO for the correction of anemia in patients with early CKD.

A second study in CKD patients not on dialysis showed the effectiveness of fixed doses of darbepoetin alfa administered SC once every other week

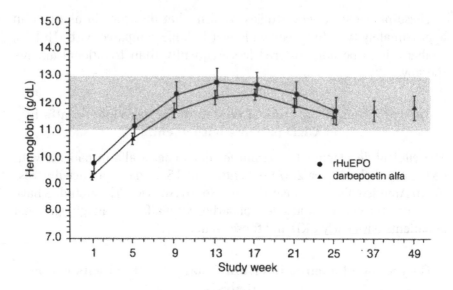

Figure 4. Mean (95% confidence interval) hemoglobin concentrations at 4-week intervals after treatment with rHuEPO and darbepoetin alfa in CKD patients not on dialysis. The shaded area indicates the target hemoglobin range [38].

for the treatment of anemia in rHuEPO-naive patients [39]. Starting with a dose of 0.75 µg/kg, the dose of darbepoetin alfa was titrated to achieve and maintain hemoglobin within the target range of 11.0–13.0 g/dl. An interim analysis of the initial 23 patients enrolled into the study showed that the median time to achieve a hemoglobin response was 6 weeks (range: 0–17 weeks) and 91% of patients reached the target hemoglobin range within 10 weeks of initiating darbepoetin alfa therapy (95% confidence interval: 73.2%, 97.6%). The median darbepoetin alfa dose at the time of hemoglobin response was 50 µg every other week (range: 30–130 µg) [39].

These studies confirm that darbepoetin alfa is effective in the management of anemia in CKD patients not on dialysis when administered once-weekly or once every other week. The decreased frequency of administration relative to rHuEPO offers a genuine advantage for patients with early CKD who do not attend renal clinics on a frequent basis.

Correction of anemia in rHuEPO-naive patients on dialysis

Anemia in patients on dialysis can be effectively corrected with darbepoetin alfa at a reduced frequency relative to rHuEPO [41]. An open-label, dose-escalation study involving patients on hemodialysis treated with IV darbepoetin alfa, and another study involving patients on peritoneal dialysis receiving SC darbepoetin alfa concluded that an appropriate starting dose for the treatment of anemia in dialysis patients is 0.45–0.75 μg/kg when administered once-weekly [41]. A dose-dependent increase in hemoglobin was observed in both studies (Figure 5), with no difference between once and three times weekly dosing [42]. Darbepoetin alfa doses of 0.45 and 0.75 μg/kg/week provided optimal responses in 60–70% of patients [41].

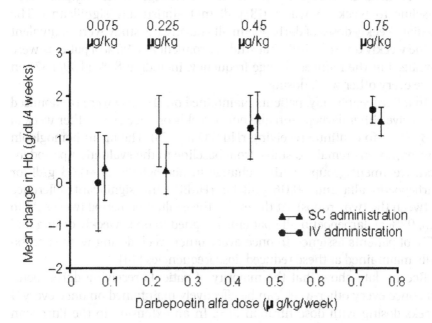

Figure 5. Mean rise in hemoglobin concentration (95% confidence interval) over the first 4 weeks of SC darbepoetin alfa administration in peritoneal dialysis patients (▲) and IV darbepoetin alfa administration in hemodialysis patients (●). Reproduced with the permission of Oxford University Press [42].

Maintenance of hemoglobin levels with darbepoetin alfa

Studies in dialysis patients with CKD who were maintained on rHuEPO showed that hemoglobin levels could be effectively maintained when patients were then randomized to darbepoetin alfa at a reduced dosing frequency (once-weekly, once every other week and once every 3 weeks) compared with rHuEPO [43–45].

An open-label study in patients on dialysis confirmed the ability of darbepoetin alfa to safely maintain hemoglobin levels for up to 1 year [35]. Patients on hemodialysis or peritoneal dialysis were switched from rHuEPO to darbepoetin alfa therapy. In patients receiving rHuEPO once-weekly ($n = 157$), the frequency of darbepoetin alfa was reduced to once every other week. In patients receiving rHuEPO twice ($n = 203$) or three times ($n = 343$) weekly, the frequency of darbepoetin alfa administration was reduced to once-weekly. The mean change in hemoglobin from baseline to week 36 was 0.08 g/dl (not statistically significant). The median weekly doses of darbepoetin alfa during the study were equivalent to the weekly dose of rHuEPO at study enrolment and 96% of patients were managed at the reduced dosage frequency, including 89% (139/157) on once every other week dosing.

In a European study, patients maintained on rHuEPO were randomized to receive either darbepoetin alfa once-weekly or once every other week ($n = 347$), or to continue receiving rHuEPO ($n = 75$). The mean hemoglobin concentrations remained stable from baseline to the evaluation period for both treatment groups, with a change in hemoglobin of –0.03 g/dl for darbepoetin alfa and –0.06 g/dl for rHuEPO (no significant difference between the two groups). At the end of the evaluation period (weeks 24 to 32), 97% of darbepoetin alfa patients assigned to once-weekly dosing and 95% of patients assigned to once every other week dosing were success-fully maintained at these reduced dose frequencies [44].

Recent data show that the majority of patients receiving darbepoetin alfa once every other week can be effectively maintained on once every 3 weeks dosing with dose titration [45]. In an extension to the European study, 34 dialysis patients with mean baseline hemoglobin between 10.0 and 13.0 g/dl and receiving darbepoetin alfa once every 2 weeks were switched to once every 3 weeks dosing to determine whether hemoglobin could be successfully maintained (within the range 10.0–13.0 g/dl) at this reduced dosing frequency. Twenty-six (76%) patients were successfully maintained on once every 3 weeks dosing. The mean change in hemoglobin from baseline to evaluation (–0.18 g/dl) was not statistically significant [45].

These studies show that darbepoetin alfa is as effective as rHuEPO for correcting and maintaining hemoglobin levels, but with the clinical advantage of less frequent dosing.

Safety profile of darbepoetin alfa

Darbepoetin alfa is well tolerated and has a comparable safety profile to that of rHuEPO [46,47]. The safety and tolerability of darbepoetin alfa was evaluated on the basis of an integrated safety database of 1598 patients who received darbepoetin alfa and 600 patients who received rHuEPO. Safety information was available for up to 1 year for most patients and a long-term safety study was used to collect safety information beyond 1 year.

Three percent of darbepoetin alfa patients and 4% of rHuEPO patients discontinued treatment due to adverse events. The percentage of deaths during the study period was 6% in both treatment groups. Cardiac-related events were the most common cause of death (3% darbepoetin alfa, 5% rHuEPO) [46,47], as would be expected in the ESRD population overall [48]. The incidence of deaths in the darbepoetin alfa clinical program was low relative to the dialysis population as a whole and the most common causes of death were as would be expected for patients with CKD [48].

Adverse events reported in clinical trials of darbepoetin alfa in CKD patients with anemia were similar to those reported with rHuEPO. The most common adverse events were hypertension, hypotension, myalgia and headache (Table 2). These events are characteristic of CKD patients and are not necessarily attributable to darbepoetin alfa or rHuEPO. The adverse events most commonly considered to be related to treatment by investigators were hypertension (9% darbepoetin alfa, 7% rHuEPO) and injection-site pain (7% darbepoetin alfa, 1% rHuEPO). Injection-site pain was generally mild and transient in nature. All other adverse events were reported with a similar incidence in both treatment groups [42].

Analyses of laboratory results showed no trends indicative of a treatment-related effect. All patients in the darbepoetin alfa clinical trial program were tested for darbepoetin alfa (and rHuEPO) antibodies. To date, there have been no reports of antibody formation associated with darbepoetin alfa in clinical trials of more than 1500 patients [42].

Darbepoetin alfa can be safely withdrawn in patients whose hemoglobin exceeds the desired upper target level. In patients with CKD and those on dialysis whose hemoglobin concentration reached over 14 g/dl, cessation of treatment resulted in a progressive reduction in hemoglobin concentration at a similar rate for both darbepoetin alfa and rHuEPO treatment

Table 2. Proportion of patients reporting adverse events (incidence >10%) [47]

	Incidence (%)	
Adverse events	Darbepoetin alfa ($n = 1598$)	rHuEPO ($n = 600$)
Body as a whole		
Peripheral edema	11	17
Cardiovascular		
Hypertension	23	26
Hypotension	22	24
CNS/PNS		
Headache	16	18
Gastrointestinal		
Diarrhea	16	21
Vomiting	15	20
Nausea	14	24
Abdominal pain	12	17
Musculoskeletal		
Myalgia	21	27
Arthralgia	11	14
Respiratory		
Upper respiratory infection	14	23
Dyspnea	12	18

groups [42]. The rate of decline of hemoglobin after withholding anemia therapy appears to be determined by the rate of loss of aging erythrocytes as they reach the end of their life span, and not by clearance of darbepoetin alfa or rHuEPO.

SUMMARY AND CONCLUSIONS

The introduction of rHuEPO for the management of anemia in CKD is certainly one of the milestones in the history of nephrology. It has dramatically improved the lives of CKD patients with anemia since its approval in 1989. Increased survival, decreased hospitalizations, improved brain and cognitive function, and improved quality of life for patients are some of the benefits witnessed by the use of rHuEPO in the treatment of anemic CKD patients.

The beneficial effects on fatigue, exercise tolerance, and the cardiovascular system are major factors contributing to the positive risk-benefit ratio of rHuEPO. Remaining clinical issues related to this compound include the requirement for frequent dosing, and predicting and overcoming resistance. The requirement for frequent administration can place a significant burden on patients with early CKD who may have to make special trips to the clinic for their injection.

Patients often require transportation to a predialysis clinic two to three times per week for their rHuEPO injection, and it is difficult for patients with certain socioeconomic stature to maintain this type of schedule. It is common that CKD patients often miss many rHuEPO doses and their persistent anemia is certainly a factor in their development of left ventricular hypertrophy.

Research into the factors and structural features that control the *in vivo* activity of EPO has led to the discovery of another revolutionary biotechnology product, darbepoetin alfa [30]. Darbepoetin alfa represents a new generation of long-acting erythropoietic proteins. It is biochemically distinct from rHuEPO, having differences in amino-acid sequence and increased sialylated carbohydrate content, which results in a prolonged half-life and enhanced biological activity. This enables the treatment of anemia in CKD patients with the advantage of less frequent dosing compared with rHuEPO [12]. Less frequent administration may improve compliance and decrease administration costs.

Studies confirm that once-weekly, and every other week, dosing with darbepoetin alfa can correct and maintain hemoglobin concentrations in CKD patients with anemia [12]. Recently published data on darbepoetin alfa suggest that hemoglobin levels can be maintained with once every 3 weeks dosing in patients receiving dialysis [45]. Experience shows that patients often require transportation to a predialysis clinic two to three times per week for their rHuEPO injection, and it is difficult for patients with certain socioeconomic stature to maintain this type of schedule.

Therefore, the decreased frequency of dosing with darbepoetin alfa may improve compliance in this patient population. Less frequent dosing potentially results in many benefits, for example fewer office visits, less transportation issues, decreased resource requirements. A reduction in patient discomfort, fewer needle sticks, and decreased risk of needle stick injury are further advantages. Frequency of administration is a genuine advantage to patients with early CKD who do not attend predialysis clinics on a frequent basis. Therefore, the less frequent administration required with darbepoetin alfa should increase utilization of anemia therapy and improve anemia management in this group of patients.

Darbepoetin alfa has recently been approved in Europe, Australia, and the US for the management of anemia in patients with CKD. With the potential of simplifying anemia management for patients and providers, darbepoetin alfa could become the new standard of care in anemia management.

REFERENCES

1. Jones CA, McQuillan G, Kusek J. Serum creatinine levels in the US population: Third National Health and Nutrition Examination Survey. Am J Kidney Dis. 1998;32:992–9. [Erratum, Am J Kidney Dis. 2000;35:178.]
2. National Institutes of Health. National Insitutes of Diabetes and Digestive and Kidney Diseases. Healthy people 2010. Chronic Kidney Disease 2000.
3. Kausz AT, Khan SS, Abichandani R, et al. Management of patients with chronic renal insufficiency in the Northeastern United States. J Am Soc Nephrol. 2001; 12:1501–7.
4. Obrador GT, Ruthazer R, Arora P, Kausz AT, Pereira BJ. Prevalence of and factors associated with suboptimal care before initiation of dialysis in the United States. J Am Soc Nephrol. 1999;10:1793–800.
5. Pereira BJ. Optimization of pre-ESRD care: the key to improved dialysis outcomes. Kidney Int. 2000;57:351–65.
6. Kuriyama S, Tomonari H, Yoshida H, Hashimoto T, Kawaguchi Y, Sakai O. Reversal of anemia by erythropoietin therapy retards the progression of chronic renal failure, especially in nondiabetic patients. Nephron. 1997;77:176–85.
7. Klang B, Bjorvell H, Clyne N. Quality of life in predialytic uremic patients. Qual Life Res. 1996;5:109–16.
8. Caro J, Brown S, Miller O, Murray T, Erslev AJ. Erythropoietin levels in uremic nephric and anephric patients. J Lab Clin Med. 1979;93:449–58.
9. Eckardt KU. Pathophysiology of renal anemia. Clin Nephrol 2000;53:S2-8.
10. Winearls CG, Oliver DO, Peppard MJ, Reid C, Downing MR, Cotes PM. Effect of human erythropoietin derived from recombinant DNA on the anaemia of patients maintained by chronic hemodialysis. Lancet. 1986;2:1175–8.
11. Eschbach JW, Egrie JC, Downing MR, Browne JK, Adamson JW. Correction of the anemia of end-stage renal disease with recombinant human erythropoietin. Results of a combined phase I and phase II clinical trial. N Engl J Med. 1987; 316:73–8.
12. Macdougall IC. Novel erythropoiesis stimulating protein. Semin Nephrol. 2000; 20:375–81.
13. Lin F-K, Suggs S, Lin CH, et al. Cloning and expression of the human erythropoietin gene. Proc Natl Acad Sci USA. 1985;82:7580–4.
14. Eschbach JW. The anemia of chronic renal failure: pathophysiology and the effects of recombinant erythropoietin. Kidney Int. 1989;35:134–48.
15. Sundal E, Kaeser U. Correction of anemia of chronic renal failure with recombinant human erythropoietin: safety and efficacy of one year's treatment in a European multicentre study of 150 haemodialysis-dependent patients. Nephrol Dial Transplantation. 1989;4:979–87.
16. Lim VS, DeGowin RL, Zavala D, et al. Recombinant human erythropoietin treatment in pre-dialysis patients. A double blind placebo-controlled study. Ann Intern Med. 1989;110:108–14.

17. Revicki D, Brown R. Health related quality of life associated with recombinant human erythropoietin therapy for predialysis chronic kidney disease patients. Am J Kidney Dis. 1995;25:548–54.

18. Moreno F, Lopez Gomez JM, Sanz-Guajardo D, Jofre R, Valderrabano F. Quality of life in dialysis patients. A Spanish multicentre study. Spanish Cooperative Renal Patients Quality of Life Study Group. Nephrol Dial Transplantation. 1996;11: 125–9.

19. Drueke T, Eckardt K, Frei U, et al. Does early anemia correction prevent complications of chronic renal failure? Clin Nephrol. 1999;51:1–11.

20. Egrie J, Eschbach JW, McGuire T, et al. Pharmacokinetics of recombinant human erythropoietin administrered in hemodialysis patients. Kidney Int. 1988;33:262.

21. Kampf D, Kahl A, Passlick J, et al. Single-dose kinetics of recombinant human erythropoietin after intravenous subcutaneous and intraperitoneal administration. Preliminary results. Contrib Nephrol. 1989;76:106–11.

22. Amgen Inc. Epogen package insert. Thousand Oaks, CA, USA; 2000.

23. Eschbach J, De Oreo P, Adamson J, et al. RHuEPO clinical practice guidelines for the treatment of anemia of chronic renal failure. Am J Kidney Dis. 1997;30: S192–240.

24. NKF-DOQI. NKF DOQI clinical practice guidelines for the treatment of chronic kidney failure. Am J Kidney Dis. 1997;30:S192–240.

25. Buckner FS, Eschbach JW, Haley NR, Davidson RC, Adamson JW. Hypertension following erythropoietin therapy in anemic hemodialysis patients. Am J Hypertens. 1990;3:947–55.

26. Vaziri ND. Mechanism of erythropoietin-induced hypertension. Am J Kidney Dis. 1999;33:821–8.

27. Bahlmann J, Schoter KH, Scigalla P, et al. Morbidity and mortality in hemodialysis patients with and without erythropoietin treatment: a controlled study. Contrib Nephrol. 1991;88:90–106.

28. Klinkmann H, Wieczorek L, Scigalla P. Adverse events of subcutaneous recombinant human erythropoietin therapy: results of a controlled multicenter European study. Artif Organs. 1993;17:219–25.

29. Besarab A, Flaharty KK, Erslev AJ, et al. Clinical pharmacology and economics of recombinant human erythropoietin in end-stage renal disease: the case for subcutaneous administration. J Am Soc Nephrol. 1992;2:1405–16.

30. Egrie JC, Browne JK. Development and characterization of novel erythropoiesis stimulating protein (NESP). Br J Cancer. 2001;84(supplement 1):3–10.

31. Egrie J, Browne J. Development and characterization of novel erythropoiesis stimualting protein (NESP). Nephrol Dial Transplantation. 2001;16(supplement 3):313.

32. Elliott SG, Lorenzini T, Strickland E, Delorme E, Egrie JC. Rational design of novel erythropoiesis stimulating protein (ARANESP): a super-sialylated molecule with increased biological activity. Blood. 2000;96:82a [abstract 352].

33. Macdougall IC, Gray SJ, Elston O, et al. Pharmacokinetics of novel erythropoiesis stimulating protein compared with epoetin alfa in dialysis patients. J Am Soc Nephrol. 1999;10:2392–5.

34. Allon M, Kleinman K, Walczyk M, et al. The pharmacokinetics of novel erythropoiesis stimulating protein (NESP) following chronic intravenous administration is time- and dose-linear. Presented at the 33rd Annual Meeting and Exposition of the American Society of Nephrology, Toronto, Canada, 2000.

35. Graf H, Lacombe J-L, Braun J, Gomes da Costa AA. Novel erythropoiesis stimulating protein (NESP) effectively maintains hemoglobin (Hgb) when administered at a reduced dose frequency compared with recombinant human erythropoietin (r-HuEPO) in ESRD patients. Presented at the 33rd Annual

Meeting and Exposition of the American Society of Nephrology, Toronto, Canada, 2000.

36. Lerner GR, Kale AS, Warady BA, et al. The pharmacokinetics of novel erythropoiesis stimulating protein (NESP) in pediatric patients with chronic renal failure (CRF) or end-stage renal disease. Presented at the 33rd Annual Meeting and Exposition of the American Society of Nephrology, Toronto, Canada, 2000.

37. Evans JH, Brocklebank JT, Bowmer CJ, Ng PC. Pharmacokinetics of recombinant human erythropoietin in children with renal failure. Nephrol Dial Transplantation. 1991;6:709–14.

38. Locatelli F, Olivares J, Walker R, et al. Novel erythropoiesis stimulating protein for treatment of anemia in chronic renal insufficiency. Kidney Int. 2001;60:741–7.

39. Suranyi M, Jackson L, Lubina J, McDermott-Vitak AD. Novel erythropoiesis stimulating protein (NESP) administered once every other week corrects anemia in patients with chronic renal insufficiency. Presented at the National Kidney Foundation Annual Meeting, San Francisco, CA, USA, 2001.

40. Walker R, Locatelli F, Olivares J, Wilkie M, European/Australian NESP Study Group. Novel erythropoiesis stimulating protein (NESP) corrects anemia in patients with chronic renal insufficiency (CRI) when administered at a reduced dose frequency relative to recombinant human erythropoietin (rHuEPO). Presented at the 10th Annual National Kidney Foundation Clinical Nephrology Meeting, Orlando, FL, USA, 2001.

41. Macdougall IC. Novel erythropoiesis stimulating protein (NESP) for the treatment of renal anaemia. J Am Soc Nephrol. 1998;9:258a–9a [abstract A1317].

42. Macdougall IC. An overview of the efficacy and safety of novel erythropoiesis stimulating protein (NESP). Nephrol Dial Transplantation. 2001;16:14–21.

43. Nissenson AR, Swan SK, Lindberg JS, et al. Novel erythropoiesis stimulating protein (NESP) safely maintains hemoglobin concentration levels in hemodialysis patients as effectively as r-HuEPO when administered once-weekly. Presented at the 33rd Annual Meeting and Exposition of the American Society of Nephrology, Toronto, Canada, 2000.

44. Vanrenterghem Y, Barany P, Mann J. Novel erythropoiesis stimulating protein (NESP) maintains hemoglobin in ESRD patients when administered once weekly or once every other week. J Am Soc Nephrol. 1999;10:270A [abstract A1365].

45. Vanrenterghem Y, Jadoul M, Foret M, Walker R, European/Australian Study Group. Novel erythropoiesis stimulating protein (NESP) administered once every 3 weeks by the intravenous or subcutaneous route maintains hemoglobin (Hb) in dialysis patients. Presented at the ASN/ISN World Congress of Nephrology, San Francisco CA, USA, 2001.

46. Amgen Inc. Aranesp™ package insert. Thousand Oaks, CA, USA; 2001.

47. Amgen Inc. Integrated summary of safety. Data on file.

48. United States Renal Data System. USRDS 1999 Annual Report. National Institute of Health, National Institutes of Diabetes and Digestive and Kidney Diseases, Bethesda, MD; 1999.

7. Normalizing hematocrit in renal failure: dangerous or desirable?

Iain C. Macdougall

INTRODUCTION

Although erythropoietin therapy has been available for the treatment of renal anemia for over a decade, there is still no general consensus on what the appropriate target hemoglobin to aim for is in patients with this condition [1–3]. Indeed, the question as to whether the anemia should be partially or fully corrected is arguably the most debated and controversial issue in this aspect of patient management. Why is this so? If one examines the scientific evidence relating to this topic, one can find both circumstantial evidence, and also evidence from intervention clinical trials [4–11].

Much of the circumstantial evidence supports normalization of hemoglobin, and indeed intuitively one would perhaps like to think that physiologically normal hemoglobin levels are appropriate. The scientific evidence from controlled clinical trials, however, has not massively supported this argument, with the benefits being less than might be predicted. Part of the explanation for this, however, may be in the study design of the trials. Most of the evidence comes from hemodialysis patients, and too much irreversible damage may have already been present at the time of study recruitment to allow any benefits to be seen.

Thus, it is important not to extrapolate results from one cohort of patients to the renal failure population as a whole, or even to other sub-groups of patients. At the present time, and possibly due to the lack of evidence, both the NKF-DOQI Guidelines [12] and the European Best Practice Guidelines [13] do not differentiate between sub-groups of renal failure patients, and arbitrary thresholds of >11 g/dl and 11–12 g/dl, respectively have been suggested.

Onyekachi Ifudu (ed.), Renal Anemia: Conflicts and Controversies, 65–80.
© 2002 Kluwer Academic Publishers.

The aim of this article is to question firstly why we aim for subnormal hemoglobin levels, and then to review the scientific evidence gained from the clinical trials examining full versus partial correction of anemia. The concept of not using the same target hemoglobin for all modalities of renal failure patients will be explored, as will the concept of individualizing the target hemoglobin for a particular patient, pending results from other scientific studies.

Why do we aim for subnormal hemoglobin levels?

Ever since erythropoietin therapy was introduced as a therapeutic agent for renal anemia, clinicians have been aiming for only partial hemoglobin correction. There are several possible explanations for this. The first is historical, in that the two earliest pivotal studies from Seattle [14] and Oxford/London [15] aimed for only partial correction of anemia. This study design was then extrapolated into other clinical trial protocols, and the habit became stuck. There has also been concern that full correction of anemia in renal failure patients might expose such individuals to an increased risk of developing adverse events, such as hypertension and vascular access thrombosis, or even hypertensive encepalopathy and seizures (as seen in the earliest studies of erythropoietin).

The third explanation to consider is that the largest study ever conducted to investigate this issue (the US Normal Hematocrit Study) [4] failed to live up to the expectation that dialysis patients randomized to a normal hematocrit would have a better outcome than those aiming for a conventional (subnormal) hematocrit. Some purist nephrologists might also argue that, in the current climate of evidence-based medicine, there is no conclusive evidence that targeting a normal hematocrit in patients receiving erythropoietin results in a significant improvement in morbidity and mortality compared with partial correction of the anemia. Finally, there are significant cost considerations.

At the present time, and probably for the foreseeable future, erythropoietin remains a fairly expensive treatment. Many renal units treat large numbers of patients with erythropoietin, and the treatment is long-term. Only if the patient dies or receives a renal transplant will erythropoietin usually be stopped. The cost of fully correcting anemia is considerably greater than that of partially correcting the condition [16].

Evidence from clinical trials

(i) Dialysis patients

In retrospect, it was probably appropriate for the first two pivotal studies on anemia correction to target a subnormal hemoglobin. Many of the patients recruited to the studies in Seattle [14] and Oxford/London [15] had very severe anemia, which had been present for quite some time. With any new therapy, it is sensible to proceed cautiously, and the main aim of these two studies was to ascertain whether recombinant human erythropoietin could produce a rise in hemoglobin. At this stage, establishing efficacy and safety were the main considerations, and issues such as the optimum target hemoglobin were not a priority at this stage.

The status quo was maintained for the next 6–7 years, until Joe Eschbach presented the results of his small clinical trial of hematocrit normalization at the American Society of Nephrology Meeting in late 1993 [17]. This study involved 13 hemodialysis patients in whom the mean hematocrit was increased from 32% up to 41%. There was no control group, but there were significant further reductions in left ventricular mass, increases in exercise capacity, and improvements in some quality-of-life parameters. No significant adverse events were reported in any of the 13 patients [17].

Thus, the gauntlet for hemoglobin normalization was thrown down. Several large prospective multicenter controlled studies were then designed to examine the hypothesis that full correction of anemia might confer additional benefits for the patient (Table 1) [4–8]. The first of these was the US Normal Hematocrit Trial [4], which began in June 1994. This was a randomized prospective open-label study involving 51 centers in the USA. To enter the study, patients had to be on regular hemodialysis, and to have clinical evidence of ischemic heart disease or congestive heart failure. 1233 such patients were recruited, 618 of whom were randomized to target a hematocrit of 42% (hemoglobin around 14 g/dl) and 615 of whom were to remain at a hematocrit around 30% (hemoglobin around 10 g/dl).

The primary end-points in this study were death or first non-fatal myocardial infarction, and the intended follow-up period was three years. The study was however aborted after 29 months by the Safety Monitoring Committee. The reason for this was that there were 183 deaths in the "normal" hematocrit group compared with 150 deaths in the "conventional" hematocrit group. There were also 19 first non-fatal myocardial infarctions in the higher hematocrit group compared with 14 such events in the conventional hematocrit group (Figure 1). While this did not quite

Table 1. Studies on normalization of hemoglobin in dialysis and CKD patients

Study	Patient cohort	Study design	Outcome	Reference
US Normal Haematocrit Trial	HD patients (n = 1233)	Randomised prospective controlled	No improvement in mortality ↑ vascular access thrombosis	[4]
Scandinavian multicenter study	HD, PD, CKD patients (n = 416)	Randomized prospective controlled	No difference in mortality. ↑ Q of L.	[5,6,7]
Canadian multicentere study	HD patients (n = 159)	Randomized prospective controlled	No difference in mortality. ↑ Q of L.	[8]
Spanish ulticenter study	HD patients (n = 117)	Prospective uncontrolled	↑ Q of L	[9]
Australian study	HD patients (n = 14)	Randomized crossover	↑ exercise capacity. ↑ cardiac function ↑ Q of L.	[10,11]
Eschbach et al.	HD patients (n = 13)	Prospective uncontrolled	↑ exercise capacity. ↓ LV mass ↑ Q of L	[17]
Barany et al.	HD patients	Prospective uncontrolled	↑ exercise capacity.	[19]
Stray-Gunderson et al.	HD patients	Prospective uncontrolled	↑ exercise capacity	[20]
Hayashi et al.	CKD patients (n = 9)	Prospective uncontrolled	↓ LV mass	[23]
Berns et al.	HD patients	Prospective uncontrolled	BP stable	[26]
Conlon et al.	HD patients	Prospective uncontrolled	BP stable	[27]

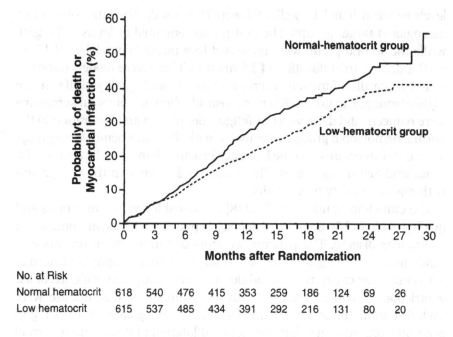

Figure 1. Kaplan-Meier estimates of the probability of death or a first nonfatal myocardial infarction in the normal-hematocrit and low-hematocrit groups.

reach statistical significance, it was borderline for this, and the statisticians concluded that the hypothesis that hemoglobin normalization would result in fewer primary end-point events could not be realized even if the study were allowed to continue [4].

It is important to remember that this study did not prove that hemoglobin normalization was dangerous, only that this practice was not of benefit in this patient population. There was also a curious paradox from this study, namely that in a *post hoc* analysis there was an inverse relationship between hematocrit and mortality in both groups of patients [18]. The explanation for this study outcome remains unclear; it is by no means certain that the hematocrit *per se* accounted for the results, and other factors, such as the greater usage of intravenous iron in the normal hematocrit group, may have been contributory. There was however a significantly greater incidence of vascular access thrombosis in the higher hematocrit group.

The Scandinavian Multicenter Trial [5–7] recruited a total of 416 patients, most of whom were on hemodialysis or peritoneal dialysis, but a few CKD patients were also included. All patients had stable hemoglobin levels between 9 and 12 g/dl, and were then randomized into one of two hemoglobin target groups. The first group remained at levels <12 g/dl, while the second group were increased to a target hemoglobin of 13.5–16.0 g/dl for a total duration of 18 months. There were modest improvements in cardiac function, exercise capacity, and quality-of-life in the higher hemoglobin group. After one year of follow up, physical symptoms were reduced, and there was less fatigue, depression and frustration in the normal hemoglobin group as compared with the lower hemoglobin group. Similar trends occurred in the Leicester Uraemic Symptoms Scale, the ADL Scale, and Self-Image scales. There was no difference in the two groups with regard to safety or mortality.

The Canadian Multicenter Trial [8] evaluated left ventricular mass and quality-of-life in 159 anemic hemodialysis patients with asymptomatic left ventricular disease. The patients were divided into two groups prior to randomization, one group had left ventricular hypertrophy and normal left ventricular cavity volume, while the other group had evidence of left ventricular dilatation. Patients with symptomatic cardiac disease were excluded from the study. Normalization of hemoglobin to 13–14 g/dl prevented progression of left ventricular dilatation in those with a normal left ventricular volume at baseline, but did not reverse pre-existing concentric left ventricular hypertrophy or left ventricular dilatation once established. Quality-of-life was also assessed in this study.

At 24 and 48 weeks, improvements in the Kidney Disease Questionnaire and SF36 Questionnaire scores were found. Normalization had the least effect in those with established left ventricular hypertrophy, and the greatest impact was in those with left ventricular dilatation. Changes in depression, fatigue, and relationships were the parameters showing the greatest effect from hemoglobin normalization.

There are also a number of uncontrolled studies examining full correction of anemia. The Spanish Multicenter Study [9] specifically examined quality-of-life issues in stable hemodialysis patients under the age of 65. The study was prospective, and follow-up was for 6 months. Patients with diabetes, previous stroke, seizures, or severe co-morbidity were excluded from the study. The hemoglobin was increased from 10.2 to 12.5 g/dl in 117 patients, and significant improvements in the Karnofsky and Sickness Impact Profile Scores were seen. There was also a reduction in the number of patients hospitalized, and in their length of hospital stay during the 6 months of the study compared with the preceding 6-month period. No safety concerns with hemoglobin normalization were found in this study.

Two studies from Australia have been reported by McMahon et al. [10,11] on the same cohort of hemodialysis patients. Although only 14 patients were recruited to these studies, the protocol utilized a scientifically robust randomized prospective cross-over design. Thus, all patients were assessed at a hemoglobin level of 10 g/dl and a hemoglobin of 14 g/dl in randomized order. There were significant improvements in exercise capacity, quality-of-life, maximum oxygen consumption, and cardiac parameters at a hemoglobin of 14 g/dl compared to 10 g/dl. Further studies by Barany et al. [19] and Stray-Gunderson et al. [20] also showed improved exercise capacity with normalization of hemoglobin compared with partial correction of anemia.

(ii) CKD patients

In contrast to dialysis patients, there are very limited data on normalization of hemoglobin in the CKD population. As will be discussed below, there may be a stronger case for fully correcting the hemoglobin in these patients who have not been exposed to anemia for such a long time, and who have never been rendered severely anemic. There is increasing interest in starting erythropoietin at an earlier stage in the development of renal failure, and indeed there is an increasing scientific rationale for doing so. We are now aware that by the time the patients start renal replacement therapy they already have a high prevalence of cardiac dysfunction [21,22].

There is one prospective study examining the cardiovascular effects of normalizing hemoglobin with erythropoietin in CKD patients. Hayashi et al. [23] assessed left ventricular mass, 24-hour blood pressure monitoring, and changes in renal function in 9 CKD patients after partial correction (target hematocrit 30%) and normalization (target hematocrit 40%) of their anemia. Left ventricular mass progressively decreased from 140.6 ± 12.1 g/m^2 at baseline, to 126.9 ± 10.0 g/m^2 after partial correction of anemia at 4 months, to 111.2 ± 8.3 g/m^2 after normalization of anemia after 12 months. There was no change in the rate of progression of renal failure over the 12 months of the study [23].

In addition, there are currently ongoing multicenter studies of erythropoietin in CKD patients in the UK, Canada, and Australia, and a global study of erythropoietin targeting two different hemoglobin concentrations in such patients has also recently been launched. The latter is the CREATE Study (Cardiovascular Reduction Early Anaemia Treatment with Epoetin beta). In group 1, patients are started on erythropoietin when their hemoglobin falls below 12.5 g/dl, and they are then treated to maintain a hemoglobin concentration between 13.0 and 15.0 g/dl. The group 2 (control) patients only start erythropoietin when their hemoglobin falls below 10.5 g/dl, and they are targeted to maintain a hemoglobin concentration between 10.5 and 11.5 g/dl.

Although it may be quite some time before any data are available from this study, it is the first one to address specifically the issue of preventing renal anemia developing in the first place, and also maintaining renal failure patients with a normal hemoglobin concentration throughout the progression of their disease. Until such data become available, however, it is difficult to make any judgements either way about normalizing hemoglobin in CKD patients. In contrast to dialysis patients, however, CKD patients do not have the problems of fluid shifts affecting the variability in hemoglobin concentration.

Individualization of target hemoglobin

The scientific data from the normalization of hemoglobin studies mentioned above make it difficult, if not impossible, to have a unifying policy for all renal failure patients with anemia. Thus, it is inappropriate to extrapolate data from a patient cohort of hemodialysis patients with known ischemic heart disease or congestive cardiac failure, to a population of young, fit CKD patients. Until further scientific data become available, therefore, it would appear that a sensible policy is to tailor the target hemoglobin to the individual requirements of the patient. To illustrate this point, I would like to present two completely contrasting fictitious cases which were deliberately selected for a previous article on this subject [16].

Case 1 is a 26-year-old man who recently reached end-stage renal failure from chronic glomerulonephritis. He has been on automated peritoneal dialysis for three months, and his hemoglobin at the time of starting dialysis was 9.2 g/dl, having been 11 g/dl four months earlier. He was started on erythropoietin therapy, and his hemoglobin was gradually increasing. He had borderline hypertension, easily controlled by a long-acting calcium antagonist, but he was otherwise very well with no other co-morbid conditions. He works as a builder, and until recently was captain of the local rugby team.

Unfortunately, his level of fitness had deteriorated to an extent that he could no longer compete at the level required of him. He had undergone a number of cardiac investigations as part of a work-up for renal transplantation; he had a normal exercise treadmill test with no signs of myocardial ischemia, and a normal echocardiogram with an ejection fraction of 56% and no evidence of left ventricular hypertrophy. What should his target hemoglobin on erythropoietin be?

Case 2 is a frail 74-year-old lady with diabetic nephropathy who has been on unit-based hemodialysis for 13 years. She was heavily transfusion-dependent when she started dialysis, but this ceased when she commenced erythropoietin therapy in 1992. She did, however, also suffer from active sero-negative rheumatoid arthritis over the years, and this had resulted in some resistance to her erythropoietin, with hemoglobin levels ranging from 7.2 to 9.9 g/dl over the last 8 years. She had suffered two myocardial infarctions in 1994 and 1997, and this had left her with a moderately severe ischemic cardiomyopathy, causing NYHA Grade III heart failure. She had two previous failed vascular access episodes, with a thrombosis of her left radial fistula in 1996, and a thrombosed left brachial fistula in 1999. She was currently dialyzing satisfactorily via a right brachial PTFE graft.

Because of her arthritis, she was largely wheelchair-bound and often breathless at rest due to her heart failure. Of late, she was becoming somewhat forgetful and intermittently confused, although she did have a supportive and caring husband. A CT scan of her brain showed changes of diffuse atherosclerotic cerebrovascular disease, but with no discreet lesion. Her family ask you what level of hemoglobin you are aiming for. What do you answer?

In brief, Case 1 is a fit young man with no significant co-morbidity who has a physically demanding job and an active life-style, whereas Case 2 is a frail elderly lady with multiple other medical problems, including significant cardiac disease and a limited life-expectancy. In real life, one has to select a target hemoglobin for each patient, but should this be the same for both patients or should it be individualized? Having a unit policy on target hemoglobin, or devising clinical guidelines on this issue, tends to consider a total population, whereas this population is made up of many different individuals who may have very different characteristics or clinical features. With reference to the two cases described above, one could offer an argument for normalizing hemoglobin in the first patient, whereas the scientific evidence [4] suggests a note of caution in doing the same for patient number 2. There are quite a number of factors that may influence the choice of target hemoglobin in an individual patient (Table 2), and these will be discussed in turn.

Table 2. Factors affecting choice of target hemoglobin in an individual patient

---

Age
Gender
Occupation
Level of physical activity
Length of time with chronic renal failure/renal anemia
Starting hemoglobin/length of time on epoetin
Co-morbid conditions
Dialysis modality

Age

There are no studies specifically looking at the choice of target hemoglobin in the elderly versus the younger population. We do know that elderly patients benefit from epoetin therapy both with regard to their exercise capacity [10] and cardiac function [24]. There are, however, two reasons why the Nephrologist uses erythropoietin therapy: firstly for a fairly rapid improvement in anemic symptoms, exercise capacity, and quality-of-life, and secondly to improve cardiac function along with (hopefully) long-term survival. Whilst the first of these criteria is applicable to patients of all ages, the potential impact of the latter phenomenon is clearly much greater in younger patients than in the frail elderly patient whose life-expectancy is less than two years. More aggressive anemia management may therefore be more appropriate in the younger patient.

Gender

Again, few studies have differentiated between males and females in terms of target hemoglobin. Interestingly, the Scandinavian Multicenter Study [5–7] did aim for a higher target hemoglobin in male patients (14.5–16.0 g/dl) compared to females (12.5–14.0 g/dl), but there was no gender difference in either the US Normal Hematocrit Trial [4] or the Canadian Multicenter Study [8]. In healthy individuals, there is a higher physiological hemoglobin in males compared to females, although this becomes less marked when the latter become post-menopausal. Some might argue that this physiological difference between males and females should be maintained in renal failure patients; others might suggest that most female dialysis patients are post-menopausal, either due to age or to biological factors causing premature menopause in uraemic patients. If one were to select a target hemoglobin for a fit and healthy male hemodialysis patient aged 25 years vs. a fit and healthy female dialysis patient aged 25 years who is still menstruating, then there may be some rationale in selecting a slightly lower target hemoglobin concentration for the latter patient. Much of this discussion is, however, speculative with little in the way of scientific data to support it.

Occupation

If a young patient is in full-time employment, and particularly if the job involves fairly strenuous physical activity, then there may be a rationale for maximizing exercise capacity in these patients. There is indeed evidence that physical capacity and maximum oxygen consumption is greater in dialysis patients with a hemoglobin concentration of around 14 g/dl compared with one around 10 g/dl [10]. This is true for both young and old patients.

Level of physical activity

For the same reasons as indicated in the previous section, a patient with a fairly active life-style involving much physical activity (including sport) would benefit from a higher rather than a lower hemoglobin.

Length of time with chronic renal failure/renal anemia

It is well-known that physiological homeostatic mechanisms, such as altered diphosphoglycerate levels (causing a shift in the oxygen dissociation curve), come into play during chronic anemia. It is these compensatory mechanisms that allow a patient with homozygous sickle cell disease to function fairly well with a hemoglobin concentration of around 5–6 g/dl between blood transfusions. The length of time a patient has suffered from renal anemia, and indeed the severity of this condition, may influence the potency and reversibility of these compensatory mechanisms.

Thus, if a patient has been exposed to a hemoglobin of between 6 and 8 g/dl for several years, homeostatic mechanisms may have become so established that to bring the hemoglobin concentration up to 14 g/dl in the space of a few months might be deleterious. It may in fact result in "relative" polycythemia for such patients, and this may also explain why severely anemic patients previously developed hypertensive encephalopathy or seizures even with a sub-optimal hemoglobin. Conversely, if a patient has been exposed to anemia for a short time (as illustrated in Case 1) then they may be better equipped to deal with a normal physiological hemoglobin level.

Starting hemoglobin/length of time on erythropoietin

For the same reasons as outlined in the previous section, both the starting hemoglobin concentration and the length of time the patient has been on erythropoietin therapy, may influence how well the patient can cope with normalization of hemoglobin. Thus, if the anemia has been mild and the patient has been on erythropoietin for several years, then the further increment in increasing their hemoglobin to normal might be achieved relatively easily. Conversely, if the hemoglobin has been increased fairly rapidly from around 7 g/dl up to 11 g/dl with erythropoietin, then a further increase to 14 g/dl might be more hazardous.

Co-morbid conditions

Conditions that may influence the choice of target hemoglobin might include cardiac disease, cerebrovascular disease, and other arteriopathic conditions, diabetes mellitus, chronic obstructive pulmonary disease, and precarious or precious vascular access (particularly if there has been a previous thrombosis). Patients with known ischemic heart disease or cardiac failure may be no better (or even worse off) with normalization of their hemoglobin compared to partial correction of anemia [4]. Although this study may have its limitations [18], one cannot ignore the findings of this large randomized controlled trial, one of the major conclusions of which was that patients with cardiac disease should not have their hemoglobin normalized until any further data become available.

There have been studies of erythropoietin therapy in diabetic patients, although no useful information has appeared on what the optimal target hemoglobin is in such patients. In view of the known microvascular disease occurring in diabetics, however, there is a rheological argument for running such patients with a slightly lower hemoglobin to reduce whole blood viscosity and improve red cell fluidity.

Non-uraemic patients with chronic obstructive pulmonary disease often develop a secondary polycythemia to compensate for chronic hypoxia. Such patients often feel less breathless with a higher hemoglobin, and there is no reason why the same rationale should not be applied to renal failure patients. There is indeed a peritoneal dialysis patient in our unit who has chronic bronchiolitis due to rejection in his heart-lung trans-plant, and who feels symptomatically less breathless at a hemoglobin of 14 g/dl than when it is reduced to 12 g/dl.

Finally, there is some evidence from controlled studies that a higher hemoglobin concentration may exacerbate the risk of a vascular access thrombosis [4,25]. The incidence of access thrombosis was higher in the initial Canadian Multicenter Study [25] in the group of patients randomized to a hemoglobin of 11.5–13.0 g/dl (7 of 38 patients) compared with those randomized to the lower hemoglobin group (9.5–11.0 g/dl; 4 of 40 patients).

Similarly in the US Normal Hematocrit Trial there was an excess of vascular access thrombosis in the patients assigned to the normal hematocrit group compared to those remaining on the lower (conventional) hematocrit (39% vs. 29%; $p = 0.001$) [4]. The implication of these data may seem somewhat obvious, but patients with a history of vascular access complications, or those with a poor quality access, or those in whom limited sites remain for further vascular access, should probably not aim for complete correction of anemia unless there are compelling reasons to do so.

Dialysis modality

As already discussed, there may be a case for targeting a different hemoglobin concentration in a pre-dialysis compared to a dialysis patient. The other issue to consider is whether the same target hemoglobin concentration should be used in hemodialysis compared with peritoneal dialysis patients. There is one important point in this respect, which is that the hemoglobin concentration in peritoneal dialysis patients is generally much more stable than in hemodialysis patients. Data shown below indicate that the hemoglobin concentration can increase by 1–3 g/dl across a dialysis session, depending on how much fluid is removed (Figure 2). Thus there might be less concern in maintaining a peritoneal dialysis patient with a hemoglobin of 14 g/dl compared with a hemodialysis patient whose pre-dialysis hemoglobin was 14 g/dl and whose post-dialysis hemoglobin was 17 g/dl.

CONCLUSIONS

The remit of this article was to question whether normalization of hemoglobin is dangerous or desirable. The body of scientific evidence does not suggest that it is particularly dangerous. Only the US Normal Hematocrit Trial suggested a borderline increase in mortality, but this was not statistically significant [4]. It is important to remember that this study, although scientifically very robust in its design, recruited only hemodialysis patients with significant cardiac disease. It is inappropriate

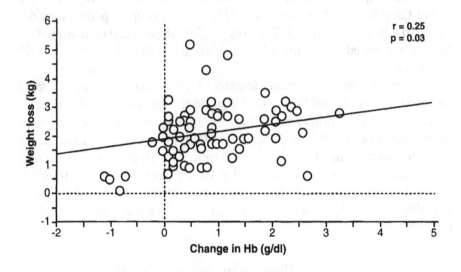

Figure 2. Change in hemoglobin concentration across dialysis (post-dialysis minus pre-dialysis sample) in relation to weight loss in a cohort of hemodialysis patients.

to extrapolate the findings to peritoneal dialysis or CKD patients, particularly in those with no cardiac dysfunction. However, neither the Scandinavian [5–7] nor the Canadian multicenter trials [8] showed any risks or adverse effects of normalizing hemoglobin in patients without symptomatic cardiac disease.

Although there was a greater incidence of vascular access thrombosis in the normalized hematocrit group, this finding was not confirmed in the Canadian multicenter study published last year [8]. Normalization of hemoglobin does not appear to have any negative impact on blood pressure stability [26,27]. The other question posed was whether hemoglobin normalization was desirable. There is certainly evidence from the studies quoted earlier that full correction of anemia may maximize the improvements in quality-of-life, cardiac function, and exercise capacity. This has to be weighed against the negative results of the US Normal Hematocrit Trial which did not show benefit. It is also apparent that to fully correct the anemia requires considerably more erythropoietin than with partial correction of anemia.

To justify normalizing hemoglobin in every renal failure patient at the present time, therefore, would not seem desirable. In selected patients, however, full correction of anemia may be both desirable and safe. Until further data become available, a sensible approach is to individualize the target hemoglobin according to the needs of the patient.

REFERENCES

1. Nissenson AR, Besarab A, Bolton WK. Target haematocrit during erythropoietin therapy. Nephrol Dial Transplantation. 1997;12:1813–16.
2. Ritz E, Amann K. Optimal haemoglobin during treatment with recombinant human erythropoietin. Nephrol Dial Transplantation. 1998;13(supplement 2): 16–22.
3. Jacobs C. Normalization of haemoglobin: why not? Nephrol Dial Transplantation. 1999;14(supplement 2):75–9.
4. Besarab A, Kline Bolton W, Browne JK, Egrie JC, Nissenson AR, Okamoto DM, Schwab SJ, Goodkin DA. The effects of normal as compared with low hematocrit values in patients with cardiac disease who are receiving hemodialysis and epoetin. N Engl J Med. 1998;339:584–90.
5. Furuland H, Linde T, Danielson BG. Cardiac function in patients with end-stage renal disease after normalization of hemoglobin with erythropoietin. J Am Soc Nephrol. 1998;9:337A.
6. Furuland H, Linde T, Danielson BG. Physical exercise capacity in patients with end-stage renal disease after normalization of hemoglobin with erythropoietin. J Am Soc Nephrol. 1998;9:337A.
7. Stombom U, Ahlmen J, Danielson B. The Scandinavian Erythropoietin Study: effects on quality of life of normalizing hemoglobin levels in uremic patients. J Am Soc Nephrol. 1999;10:142.
8. Foley RN, Parfrey PS, Morgan J, Barre PE, Campbell P, Cartier P, Coyle D, Fine A, Handa P, Kingma I, Lau CY, Levin A, Mendelssohn D, Muirhead N, Murphy B, Plante RK, Posen G, Wells GA. Effect of hemoglobin levels in hemodialysis patients with asymptomatic cardiomyopathy. Kidney Int. 2000;58:1325–35.
9. Moreno F, Sanz-Guajardo D, Lopez-Gomez JM, Jofre R, Valderrabano F. Increasing the hematocrit has a beneficial effect on quality of life and is safe in selected hemodialysis patients. Spanish Cooperative Renal Patients Quality of Life Study Group of the Spanish Society of Nephrology. J Am Soc Nephrol. 2000;11:335–42.
10. McMahon LP, McKenna MJ, Sangkabutra T, Mason K, Sostaric S, Skinner SL, Burge C, Murphy B, Crankshaw D. Physical performance and associated electrolyte changes after haemoglobin normalization: a comparative study in haemodialysis patients. Nephrol Dial Transplantation. 1999;14:1182–7.
11. McMahon LP, Mason K, Skinner SL, Burge CM, Grigg LE, Becker GJ. Effects of haemoglobin normalization on quality-of-life and cardiovascular parameters in end-stage renal failure. Nephrol Dial Transplantation. 2000;15:1425–30.
12. NKF-DOQI Work Group. NKF-DOQI clinical practice guidelines for the treatment of anemia of chronic renal failure. Am J Kidney Dis. 1997;30(supplement 3): S192–S240.
13. European Best Practice Guidelines for the management of anaemia in patients with chronic renal failure. Nephrol Dial Transplantation. 1999;14(supplement 5):1–50.

14. Eschbach JW, Egrie JC, Downing MR, Browne JK, Adamson JW. Correction of the anaemia of end-stage renal disease with recombinant human erythropoietin. N Engl J Med. 1987;316:73-8.
15. Winearls CG, Oliver DO, Pippard MJ, Reid C, Downing MR, Cotes PM. Effect of human erythropoietin derived from recombinant DNA on the anaemia of patients maintained by chronic haemodialysis. Lancet. 1986;i:1175-8.
16. Macdougall IC. Should the hematocrit be normalized in dialysis and in pre-ESRD patients? Blood Purif. 2001;19:157-67.
17. Eschbach JW, Glenny R, Robertson T, Guthrie M, Rader B, Evans R, Chandler W, Davidson R, Easterling T, Denney J, Schneider G. Normalizing the hematocrit in hemodialysis patients with EPO improves quality of life and is safe. J Am Soc Nephrol. 1993;4:425.
18. Macdougall IC, Ritz E. The Normal Haematocrit Trial in dialysis patients with cardiac disease: are we any the less confused about target haemoglobin? Nephrol Dial Transplantation. 1998;13:3030-3.
19. Barany P, Svedenhag J, Katzarski K, Divino Filno J, Norman R, Freyshuss U, Bergström J. Physiologic effects of correcting anemia in hemodialysis patients to a normal hemoglobin concentration. J Am Soc Nephrol. 1996;7:1472.
20. Stray-Gunderson J, Sams B, Goodkin D, Holloway D, Wang C, Thompson J. Improvement in functional capacity in dialysis patients with regular exercise and correction of anemia. J Am Soc Nephrol. 1997;8:112A.
21. Foley RN, Parfrey PS, Harnett JD, Kent GM, Martin CJ, Murray DC, Barre PE. Clinical and echocardiographic disease in patients starting end-stage renal disease therapy. Kidney Int. 1995;47:186-92.
22. Levin A, Thompson CR, Ethier J, Carlisle EJF, Tobe S, Mendelssohn D, Burgess E, Jindal K, Barrett B, Singer J, Djurdjev O. Left ventricular mass index increase in early renal disease: impact of decline in hemoglobin. Am J Kidney Dis. 1999;34: 125-34.
23. Hayashi T, Suzuki A, Shoji T, Togawa M, Okada N, Tsubakihara Y, Imai E, Hori M. Cardiovascular effect of normalizing the hematocrit level during erythropoietin therapy in predialysis patients with chronic renal failure. Am J Kidney Dis. 2000; 35:250-6.
24. Martinez-Vea A, Bardaji A, Garcia C, Ridao C, Richart C, Oliver JA. Long-term myocardial effects of correction of anemia with recombinant human erythro-poietin in aged patients on hemodialysis. Am J Kidney Dis. 1992;19:353-7.
25. Canadian Erythropoietin Study Group. Association between recombinant human erythropoietin and quality of life and exercise capacity of patients receiving haemodialysis. Br Med J. 1990;300:573-8.
26. Berns JS, Rudnick MR, Cohen RM, Bower JD, Wood BC. Effects of normal hematocrit on ambulatory blood pressure in epoetin-treated hemodialysis patients with cardiac disease. Kidney Int. 1999;56:253-60.
27. Conlon PJ, Kovalik E, Schumm D, Minda S, Schwab SJ. Normalization of hematocrit in hemodialysis patients with cardiac disease does not increase blood pressure. Renal Failure. 2000;22:435-44.

8. Do race, gender or mode of dialysis modulate erythropoietin response?

Barbara G. Delano

The introduction of erythropoietin (EPO) for the anemia of renal failure has clearly been one of the most important clinical advances in the treatment of end stage renal disease (ESRD). The benefits attributed to EPO use include improvement in cardiac function [1], quality of life [2], cognitive function [3] and increased sexual functioning [4] among others. To accrue these benefits, the hematocrit level is "targeted" to be between 33–36 vols % [5].

There is a disparity in the hematocrit level of dialysis patients. In general Blacks and women have a lower hematocrit than Whites and men. In a national sample of seven thousand hemodialysis patients, 47% of Blacks and 33% of Whites had a hematocrit less than the recommended target of 33 vols %. In addition, more women than men fell below this level (47% vs. 40% respectively), despite the use of larger doses of EPO [6].

ESRD treatment is expensive. It is estimated that the cost to Medicare will be 28.3 billion dollars by the year 2010 [7]. Part of these costs include payment for erythropoietin. The cost to Medicare for EPO was $842.2 million dollars in 1997 [8]. Recent United States Renal Data Systems (USRDS) data show that in patients with higher hematocrits, overall costs are actually lower [9], thus investigations as to how to achieve the target hematocrit in the most cost effective way are warranted. Any under-standings of the variables that account for individual responses to EPO are important. In this paper, we will review whether or not gender, race, mode or frequencies of dialysis modulate the response to EPO.

Does gender matter?

Women start dialysis with a lower mean hematocrit then men [6] and continue to have a lower hematocrit when they are on dialysis. Possible explanations for these differences include the following: women may

Onyekachi Ifudu (ed.), Renal Anemia: Conflicts and Controversies, 81–88.
© 2002 Kluwer Academic Publishers.

receive worse medical care: have more blood loss than men (although significant menstrual blood loss is unlikely as most women on dialysis are either menopausal or amenorrheic): have fewer androgens which are known bone marrow stimulants: respond to, or metabolize EPO differently then men. Finally women may handle iron differently.

To examine the question of differences in the quality or availability of health care for women, Daumit et al. studied almost five thousand patients with chronic renal failure who underwent invasive cardiac procedures before and after they started dialysis. Among the variables in this logistic regression analysis were socioeconomic status, medical insurance and employment. At baseline, before ESRD, women had less medical coverage and were a third less likely to have a cardiovascular procedure, but by one year of dialysis (and universal Medicare coverage) the odds ratio for the procedure was the same as for men. They concluded that provision of insurance can equalize access to care for women [10].

Madore [11], examining data from almost twenty two thousand prevalent hemodialysis patients in 1993 found that women had a mean hemoglobin that was 2.4 g/L lower than men after adjusting for iron, ferritin and EPO dose despite having insurance for dialysis. More recently, Ifudu et al. [12] in a retrospective study of 309 dialysis patients found that women required a 39% higher dose of EPO to achieve the same hematocrit as men (36 vols %) even though women were "better dialyzed" as measured by a higher mean urea reduction rate and receiving equivalent amounts of intravenous iron replacement. Goodnough [13] studied the response to blood loss in 71 non-anemic, non-uremic autologous blood donors scheduled for orthopedic surgery, who had phlebotomies and received either placebo or EPO in varying doses. They found no difference in the EPO-stimulated red blood cell volume by gender. Although non-anemic, non-uremic men and women may respond in the same way to EPO, in uremic patients data suggests that gender does make a difference. Whether this is due to hormonal or other difference is not known.

Does race matter?

Blacks start ESRD with a hematocrit that is considerably lower than Whites, and once they are on dialysis they are more likely to have a lower hematocrit whether they are on peritoneal dialysis [14], or hemodialysis [15]. Socioeconomic factors may play a role. Ifudu has shown that the relative risk for late referral of Blacks to a nephrologist is 5.6 times that of Whites [16], suggesting that pre-dialysis prescribing and monitoring of EPO is less likely to occur.

Thamer and co-workers examined prescribing practices of EPO retrospectively for 413 hemodialysis patients in 15 for-profit dialysis units in the Chicago area. Important predictors of higher initial EPO dose were the initial hematocrit and white race. These authors suggest that Blacks may be less likely to afford the 20% co-pay required for the medication [17].

The NHANES II study of 27,803 "normal" men and women found that Blacks had a mean hemoglobin that was 8.4 g/L and 5.3 g/L lower than whites, respectively. These differences were not explained by age, income, parity, oral iron intake, transferrin or ferritin. They suggest there may be racial differences in the utilization of iron or genetic differences [18].

Indeed in an interesting paper Vasquez et al. found that black renal transplant recipients required higher doses of steroids, cyclosporine, tacrolimus and mycophenolate mofetil to achieve rejection rates comparable to others. Clinical response to early rejection was achieved in 74% of Blacks and 91% of others with the same dose of steroids [19]. Black patients appear to be less responsive to ACE inhibitors [20], and in one study of regional and racial differences in response to antihypertensive medications, Blacks were less likely than Whites to achieve treatment success rates with atenolol ($p = 0.02$) or prazosin ($p = 0.03$), but were more likely to have successful control of blood pressure than whites with diltiazem ($p = 0.05$) [21].

Frackoewicz et al. conducted a 30-year MEDLINE search identifying racial differences in response to antipsychotic medications. Based on their analysis, they suggest four possible reasons for ethnic differences in response to drugs: 1) Differences due to genetic polymorphism of cytochrome P450 isoenzmes that could interfere with drug metabolism; 2) Differences in smoking, alcohol use and other drug or environmental exposure may cause differences in elimination rates; 3) Ethnic differences may exist in the number of, or affinity for drug receptors; and 4) Prescribing practices may vary. Blacks may be more likely to have lower doses prescribed or be misdiagnosed [22]. The role that these factors play in the lower hematocrit or response to EPO seen in Blacks compared to Whites remains to be determined.

Does type of dialysis matter?

In the pre EPO era, patients who were undergoing peritoneal dialysis were reported to have a better hematocrit than those undergoing hemodialysis [23]. Postulated reasons, supported by data, included a decrease in plasma volume without a change in red cell mass as found by Mehta and coworker in a study of ten CAPD patients followed for one year [24] and an increase in endogenous EPO as found by Zappacosta in four of nine patients treated with CAPD for a year [25]. It was well documented that CAPD patients required fewer blood transfusions than those on hemodialysis [26] and when patients changed therapies, moving from hemodialysis to CAPD they frequently had an increase in hematocrit [27]. The earlier literature did not pay attention to iron replacement, iron stores or amount of dialysis.

There have been several studies comparing differences in hematocrit or EPO dose required between the two dialytic therapies since the drug has become widely used. Page and House compared 157 hemodialysis and 126 peritoneal dialysis patients. Demographic data was similar in both groups. Iron stores and measures of dialysis adequacy were the same. While the mean hematocrit was equal in the two groups, 10.5 g/dl in the hemodialysis group and 10.7 g/dl in the peritoneal dialysis group, the hemodialysis patients required a significantly higher mean weekly EPO dose (7370 vs. 5790 units, $p = 0.01$).

In addition, peritoneal dialysis patients required fewer blood transfusions per month then hemodialysis patients, (RR = 0.57, 95% confidence interval 0.35–0.92), and because of this there was an annual cost difference of $2105 Canadian dollars per patient [28]. Sezer converted 34 patients from hemodialysis to peritoneal dialysis and found a significant increase in hematocrit from 10.6 ± 1.5 g/dl to 11.8 ± 1.7 g/dl, $p = 0.01$, while the serum ferritin level was significantly less ($p = 0.004$) and the weekly EPO dose decreased from 9147 ± 3862 to 5000 ± 3820 units, $p = 0.001$ [29].

Possible reasons for lower EPO requirements in peritoneal dialysis patients compared to hemodiaylsis include volume differences and higher endogenous EPO levels. In addition, no blood is lost during the dialysis procedure and there may be better clearance of "middle molecules" or inhibitors of erythropoiesis with peritoneal dialysis.

A final consideration is that there is better retention of the patients own residual renal function. Lopez-Menchero et al. analyzed the impact of residual renal function on 37 ESRD patients treated with CAPD and found that residual renal function was the most important factor in hemoglobin levels in those patients [30]. The degree of residual renal function may improve blood count because it adds to the adequacy of dialysis. Opatrny, Opatrna, Sefrna and Wirth found a significant correlation between the hematocrit level and total weekly Kt/V index in 22 patients. The mean hematocrit in 15 patients with a total weekly Kt/V (tKt/V) of less than 2.3 was $28.9 \pm 1.2\%$, while in seven patients with a tKt/V of greater than 2.3, it was $35.1 \pm 1.9\%$, $p < 0.01$ [31]. This is similar to the important observation made by Ifudu, et al, that increasing the Kt/V in hemodialysis can improve responsiveness to EPO [32].

Does frequency of dialysis matter?

Recently there has been much interest in varying dialysis schedules and times. The two most common novel approaches being evaluated are short daily hemodialysis (SDHD) which occurs for 1.5 to 2.5 hours, five or six days per week, and nocturnal home hemodialysis (NHHD), which is performed five to seven days per week for about 6–8 hours [33]. Many benefits have been proclaimed to accrue to patients undergoing more frequent dialysis including an improvement in anemia. Table 1, adapted from the paper by Lacson and Diaz-Buxo [33], shows the changes in hematological parameters reported by several experiments of more frequent dialysis. A small number of early studies of "frequent" dialysis in the pre EPO era suggested that more treatment was one way to increase hematocrit in renal failure patients.

Table 1. Anemia parameter with SDH and NHHD

Study/year	Type/# pts	Months	% change Hct or Hgb	p-Value
Bouncristiani (1988)	SDH/12	27	+70	<0.05
Bouncristiani (1997)	SDH/50	12	+17	<0.01
Lugon (1997)	SDH/5	6	+13	NS
Ting (1998)	SDH/6	6	+7.5	0.047
Pinciaroli (1999)	SDH/22	12	+35	NA
Pierratos (1998)	NHHD/12	12	+9.9	NS
Kooistra (1999)	SDH/13	6	0	NS

SDH = short daily hemodialysis, NHHD = nocturnal home hemodialysis, NS = not significant, NA = not available
Adapted from Lacson and Diaz-Buxo [33]

Bonomimi in 1972 had six patients on five treatments a week and found that the mean hematocrit rose from 16.3 to 23.8 vols % and the number of transfusions required by the patients declined [34]. Similarly, in 1988 Bouncristiani found a significant increase in the hematocrit of patients undergoing daily dialysis [35]. As reported by the NIH task force on daily dialysis, 50 patients dialyzed daily in Perugia for one year had an increase in mean hematocrit from 27–31 vols %, $p = 0.001$, while the EPO dose was reduced or discontinued. Thirteen patients in the Netherlands had no change in EPO dose or hematocrit, however they became iron deficient. The 35 patients in Mountain View, California maintained a stable hematocrit while their EPO dose was significantly reduced, and in Lyon, France, 15 patients had an increase in hemoglobin while the mean EPO dose decreased from 4000 to 1000 units/week. Patients undergoing nocturnal daily dialysis had similar results. Fifty-two patients in Toronto were able to reduce their EPO by 40% and the 22 patients in Lynchburg, Virginia also had a similar reduction in EPO requirements [36].

While in most studies of more frequent dialysis the blood count remains the same or rises with less EPO, the question is, is this do to different handling or metabolism of EPO or just the effect of "better dialysis" and the removal of an inhibitor of red cell metabolism? Ifudu's study suggests that it is the latter [32].

SUMMARY

In summary, there is much variability in hematocrit levels of ESRD patients undergoing hemodialysis and the reasons are not clear. It is known that women and Blacks start hemodialysis with a lower hematocrit level than men and Whites respectively, and this may reflect differences in predialysis care. Why these two groups don't achieve parity in hematocrits is not known, particularly since, at least in some studies, women appear to be receiving the same or more adequate dialysis, as measured by Kt/V. Both peritoneal dialysis and increased frequency of hemodialysis appear to be EPO sparing, which may reflect better removal of inhibitory substances of erythropoiesis. At the present time, we can try to optimize pre dialysis treatment of anemia, aim for excellent adequacy and continue to investigate other factors to help us understand these differences.

REFERENCES

1.   Pascual J, Teruel JL, Moya JL, Liano F, Jiminez-Mena M, Ortuno J. Regression of left ventricular hypertrophy after partial correction of anemia with erythropoietin in patients on hemodialysis: A prospective study. Clin Nephrol. 1991;35:280–7.
2.   Delano BG. Improvements in quality of life following treatment with r-HurEPO in anemic hemodialysis patients. Am J Kidney Dis. 1989;14:S14–18.

3. Wolcott DL, Marsh JT, La Rue A, Carr C, Nissenson AR. Recombinant human erythropoietin treatment may improve quality of life and cognitive function in chronic hemodialysis patients. Am J Kidney Dis. 1989;14:478–85.

4. Schaefer RM, Kobot F, Heidland A. Impact of recombinant erythropoietin in sexual potency in hemodialysis patients: Contrib Nephrol. 1989;76:273–82.

5. NKF/DOQI Guidelines. Am J Kidney Dis. 2001;37:S186–7.

6. Sehgal AR. Outcomes of renal replacement therapy among blacks and women. Am J Kidney Dis. 2000;35:S148–52.

7. US Renal Data System. USRDS 2000 Annual Data Report. Bethesda, MD, National Institutes of Health, National Institute of Diabetes and Digestive and Kidney Diseases, 2000.

8. Greer JW, Milam RA, Eggers PW. Trends in use, cost and outcomes of human recombinant erythropoietin, 1989–1998. Health Care Finance Rev. 1999;20:55–62.

9. Collins AJ, Li S, Ebben J, Ma JZ, Manning W. Hematocrit levels and associated Medicare expenditures. Am J Kidney Dis. 2000;36:282–93.

10. Daumit GL, Herman JA, Powe NR. Relation of gender and health insurance to cardiovascular procedure use in persons with progression of chronic renal disease. Med Care. 2000;38:354–65.

11. Madore F, Lowrie EG, Brugnara C, et al. Anemia in hemodialysis patients: variables affecting this outcome predictor. J Am Soc Nephrol. 1997; 8:1921–9.

12. Ifudu O, Uribarri J, Rajwant I, et al. Gender modulates responsiveness to recombinant erythropoietin. Am J Kidney Dis. 2001;38:518–22.

13. Goodnough LT, Price TH, Parvin CA. The endogenous erythropoietin response and the erythropoietic response to blood loss anemia: the effects of age and gender. J Lab Med. 1995;126:57–64.

14. Rocco MV, Frankenfield DL, Frederick PR, Pugh J, McClellan WM, Owen WF. Intermediate outcomes by race and ethnicity in peritoneal dialysis patients: results from the 1997 ESRD Core Indicator Project. National ESRD Core Indicators Workgroups. Perit Dial Int. 2000;20:328–35.

15. 2000 Annual Report ESRD Clinical Performance Measures Project. Am J Kidney Dis. 2001;37:S28.

16. Ifudu O, Dawood M, Iofel Y, Valcourt JS, Friedman EA. Delayed referral of black, hispanic and older patients with chronic renal failure. Am J Kidney Dis. 1999;33: 728–33.

17. Thamer M, Richard CM, Klingmann J, Ivanovich P, Lang G, Cotter DJ. Use of clinical guideline for treatment of anemia among hemodialysis patients. Artif Organs. 2000;24:91–4.

18. Perry GS, Byers T, Yip R, Margen, S. Iron nutrition does not account for the hemoglobin difference between Blacks and Whites. J Nutrition. 1992; 122:1417–24.

19. Vasques EM, Beneditti A. Ethnic differences in clinical response to corticosteroid treatment of acute renal allograft rejection. Transplantation. 2001; 71:229–33.

20. Matthew HW. Racial, ethnic and gender differences in response to medicines. Drug Metabol Drug Interact. 1995;12:77–91.

21. Cushman WC, Reda, DJ, Perry HM, Williams D, Abjellatif M, Materson BJ. Regional and racial differences in response to antihypertensive medication use in a randomized controlled trial of men with hypertension in the United States. VA Cooperative Study Group on Antihypertensive Agents. Arch Intern Med. 2000;27:825–31.

22. Frackiewicz EJ, Samek JJ, Herrera JM, Kurtz NM, Cutler NR. Ethnicity and antipsychotic response. Ann Pharmacother. 1997;31:1360–9.

23. Bargman JM, Oreopoulos DG. Complications other than peritonitis or those related to the catheter and the fate of uremic organ dysfunction in patients receiving peritoneal dialysis. In: KD Nolph (ed.), Peritoneal Dialysis, Kluwer Academic Publisher, Boston, p 299. 1989.
24. Mehta BR, Mogridge C, Bell JD. Changes in red cell mass, plasma volume and hematocrit in patients on CAPD. Trans Amer Soc Artif Intern Organs. 1983;29; 50–2.
25. Zappacosta AR, Carlo J, Erslev A. Normalization of hematocrit in patients with ESRD on CAPD. Am J Med. 1982;72:53–62.
26. De Paepe M, Schelstraete K, Ringoir S. Influences of continuous ambulatory peritoneal dialysis on the anemia of endstage renal disease. Kidney Int. 1983;23: 744–8.
27. Movilli E, Natale C, Cancarini G. Improvements of iron utilization and anemia in uremic patients switched from hemodialysis to continuous peritoneal dialysis. Perit Dial Bull. 1986;6:147–9.
28. Page DE, House A. Important cost differences of blood transfusions and erythropoietin between hemodialysis and peritoneal dialysis patients. Adv Perit Dial. 1998;14:87–9.
29. Sezer S, Ozdemir N, Arat Z, et al. What happens after conversion of treatment to continuous ambulatory peritoneal dialysis from hemodialysis? Adv Perit Dial. 2000;16:177–81.
30. Lopez-Menchero R, Miguel A, Garcia-Ramon R, Perez-Contreras J, Girbes V. Importance of residual renal function in CAPD: its influence on different parameters of renal replacement therapy. Nephron. 1999;83:219–25.
31. Opatrny K, Opatrna S, Sefrna F, Wirth J. The anemia in continuous ambulatory peritoneal dialysis patients is related to Kt/V index. Artif Organs. 1999;23:65–9.
32. Ifudu O, Feldman J, Friedman EA. The intensity of hemodialysis and the response to erythropoietin in patients with end-stage renal disease. N Engl J Med. 1996; 334:420–5.
33. Lacson E, Diaz-Buxo JA. Daily and nocturnal hemodialysis: How do they stack up? Am J Kidney Dis. 2001;38:225–39.
34. Bonomini V, Miolo V, Albertazzi A, Scolari P. Daily dialysis programme: Indications and results. Proc Eur Dial Transplant Assn. 1972;9:44–52.
35. Bouncristiani U, Quintaliani G, Cozzari M, Giombini LRM. Daily dialysis: long term clinical and metabolic results. Kidney Int. 1988;33:S137–40.
36. Ting G. The effects of daily dialysis on the hematocrit and blood pressure. NIH/NIDDKD Task Force on Daily Dialysis, Bethesda, MD, 2001:16–17.

9. Are uremic inhibitors of erythropoiesis clinically relevant?

Onyekachi Ifudu

INTRODUCTION

Among hemodialysis patients, low hematocrits contribute to an increased rate of hospitalizations as well as shortened survival [1,2]. Consequently, it is important that clinicians identify factors that impair response to recombinant erythropoietin (EPO) and lead to persistent anemia in hemodialysis patients.

In renal failure, anemia results mainly from diminished erythropoietin production [3]. However, in both end-stage renal disease (ESRD) and preESRD patients, there is also compelling evidence that there are substances present in serum that inhibit erythropoiesis [4–15]. The exact identity of these substances and the precise mechanism by which they exert this effect remain elusive. Candidate substances suggested to play a role in uremic inhibition of erythropoiesis include polyamines (spermidine, spermine, and putrescine), N-acetyl-seryl-aspartyl-lysyl-proline (AcSDKP), as well as some proinflammatory cytokines.

Before the emergence of EPO, studies had shown that enhanced removal of these uremic inhibitors by better dialysis ameliorates uremic anemia [13,14,16–18]. Furthermore, though the effect of dialysis adequacy on EPO responsiveness was not addressed in the original trials of EPO, several subsequent studies in ESRD patients show that enhanced removal of these uremic inhibitors of erythropoiesis improved response to EPO [19–24].

Curiously, while recent guidelines on anemia management in ESRD advocate use of intravenous iron, they omit mention of the effect of dialysis adequacy on the response to EPO as a key concern [25]. Consequently, many ESRD patients with a low hematocrit chiefly due to inadequate dialysis may inappropriately receive excess intravenous iron intended as a corrective measure. This review weighs the laboratory and clinical

Onyekachi Ifudu (ed.), Renal Anemia: Conflicts and Controversies, 89–98.
© *2002 Kluwer Academic Publishers.*

evidence underpinning a clear and significant clinical relevance of uremic inhibitors of erythropoiesis.

Scope of the problem

Though treatment with EPO has improved management of anemia in ESRD by providing an effective means for its correction, anemia persists as a significant problem in uremia therapy [26]. In ESRD patients with low hematocrit reflexly increasing the EPO dose or infusing intravenous iron is not a panacea and may not rectify the problem. In fact, while the per patient dose of EPO administered to US hemodialysis patients increased by 112 to 138% from 1990 to 1996, their maximum attained hematocrit rose by only 2 to 3 percentage points [27].

Furthermore, 44% of EPO-treated patients in the last quarter of 1997 failed to raise their hematocrit to 33% [26], the targeted treatment goal. Also, in a recent report, anemia persisted in a majority of erythropoietin-treated hemodialysis patients despite two years of continuous intravenous iron therapy [28]. Also, note worthy is the fact that the percentage of patients in each of the 18 ESRD Networks in the US with hematocrits of 33% or greater correlated inversely with the percentage of patients administered intravenous iron ($r = -0.53$; $p = 0.03$) after adjustment for dose of erythropoietin [24]. Thus, patients with low hematocrits primarily because of inadequate dialysis or other causes may inappropriately be administered excess intravenous iron intended as a corrective measure.

Resolving the issue of whether persistent anemia in many EPO-treated hemodialysis patients reflects inadequate dialysis rather than a need for additional intravenous iron has major clinical and economic implications [29]. In fact, many ESRD patients with a low hematocrit chiefly due to inadequate dialysis may inappropriately receive excess intravenous iron intended as a corrective measure [24,28]. Additionally, should better dialysis in patients not now dialyzed adequately reduce the "need" for EPO, cost-savings of hundreds of millions of dollars might result.

Laboratory studies

Both animal and human studies have found impairment of erythropoiesis in uremia attributed in part to uremic inhibitors of erythropoiesis [4–15]. However, just like the elusive uremic toxin, these inhibitors have not been consistently identified. They are purported to lie in the range of "middle-molecules" [9] and candidate substances include polyamines such as spermine and spermidine [7,11].

Other suggested uremic inhibitors of erythropoiesis include N-acetyl-seryl-aspartyl-lysyl-proline (AcSDKP), as well as some proinflammatory cytokines.

Evidence for the existence of these inhibitors and the fact that uremia suppresses erythropoiesis, include in vitro findings that uremic sera in a dose-dependent fashion inhibited the growth of human as well as murine and canine erythroid colonies [5,7,9,12,30]. Also, the inhibition of erythroid colonies by uremic sera was significantly reduced after dialytic therapy [6–8,11,12,30], suggesting extraction of inhibitors by dialysis.

Furthermore, among patients with chronic renal insufficiency (not yet on dialysis) sera from those with advanced renal failure was more effective in suppressing growth of erythroid colonies than sera from those with less severe renal failure [12]. Supporting the view that uremic serum inhibits erythropoiesis is the finding that bone marrow cells from persons with renal failure produce an amount of heme equivalent to cells from persons with normal renal function when cultured *in vitro* with erythropoietin and iron [15].

CLINICAL STUDIES

Before availability of recombinant erythropoietin

Even before the emergence of EPO, there was evidence linking anemia severity with quality of dialysis [13,14,16–18]. Clinical support for existence of uremic inhibitors of erythropoiesis included the findings that a) an infusion of erythropoietin-rich plasma from a patient with aplastic anemia resulted in reticulocytosis in normal renal function but not in severe renal failure [10], and b) anemia persisted in some patients with chronic renal failure despite high serum levels of erythropoietin (30–100 mU/ml), suggesting that erythroid cells are unable to respond to circulating erythropoietin [10,13].

Before availability of EPO, several investigators showed that uremic anemia improves with initiation of dialysis or better dialysis [13,14,16–18]. Initiation of hemodialysis therapy in some patients with chronic renal failure, or a switch from maintenance hemodialysis to continuous ambulatory peritoneal dialysis (CAPD), significantly increases the hematocrit without a concomitant increase in erythropoietin levels, suggesting enhanced extraction by dialysis of an inhibitor of erythropoiesis [13,14].

Furthermore, patients who were dialyzed thrice weekly had higher hematocrits than those dialyzed twice weekly, despite potentially more blood loss during dialysis [18], and anemia was less severe in European hemodialysis patients who received longer dialysis sessions [17].

Finally, during the seminal dialysis adequacy study of the 20th century – the National Cooperative Dialysis Study, the two groups of patients with high blood urea nitrogen had significantly lower hematocrits and greater blood transfusion requirements than their counterparts with low blood urea nitrogen levels [16].

Recombinant erythropoietin era

Several investigators reported that inadequate dialysis in patients sustained by either hemodialysis [20–24] or CAPD [31,32] is associated with a poor response to EPO (persistent low hematocrit). Also, an increase in hemodialysis dose in EPO-treated patients with low hematocrits results in an increase in their hematocrit, simultaneous with a fall in endogenous erythropoietin, suggesting enhanced removal of inhibitors of erythropoiesis [33].

Additionally, trials in both hemodialysis [34] and CAPD [35] patients discern a negative correlation between Kt/V and EPO dose – well dialyzed patients required less EPO for anemia correction than their counterparts, thereby substantially reducing cost of their care.

In fact, the strong relation between hematocrit and dialysis dose in individuals with ESRD has been corroborated by analyses of pooled data at both the dialysis facility and ESRD Network levels [20-24]. A study of all 141 hemodialysis facilities in New York State (Network 2) revealed that mean dialysis facility hematocrit correlated directly with mean dialysis facility urea reduction ratio $r = 0.32$; $p = 0.001$) [24]. Furthermore, dialysis facilities with mean urea reduction ratio greater than 70% were 3 times more likely to have a mean hematocrit above 33% (odds ratio, 3; 95 CI, 1.2 to 7.5; $p = 0.02$) than their counterparts with urea reduction ratio of 70% or less [24].

These findings are consistent with the results of the 1997 ESRD Core Indicators Project that assessed anemia management in a random sample of 7292 adult in-center hemodialysis patients in the United States [20]. The Core Indicators work group showed that patients with Kt/V <1.2 had significantly lower hematocrit compared with patients whose Kt/V was ⩾1.2 [20]. These investigators also reported a positive linear relationship between hematocrit and urea reduction ratio and observed that in their study [20], dialysis dose was a more powerful predictor of hematocrit than in prior reports.

Membrane biocompatibility and responsiveness to EPO

Findings from uncontrolled studies suggest that improved response to EPO following increased dialysis dose is due to the use of more biocompatible or high flux dialysis membranes, and not to enhanced removal of uremic inhibitors [36]. Results from recent randomized studies have disproved this notion [34,37].

Locatelli et al. [37], in a multicenter randomized controlled trial found no difference in hemoglobin level increase between patients treated for 3 months with a high-flux biocompatible membrane in comparison with those treated with a standard membrane. Also, Movilli et al. [34], in a study of 68 stable hemodialysis patients found that Kt/V exerts a significant sparing effect on EPO requirement independent of the use of biocompatible synthetic membranes.

Dialysis adequacy and endogenous erythropoietin

The relative contribution of endogenous erythropoietin to red blood cell production in patients with ESRD, with or without concomitant injections of EPO, is unknown. Though end-stage kidneys still retain the capacity to produce erythropoietin [38,39], serum endogenous erythropoietin levels do not correlate with hematocrit in ESRD [21].

Morris and Coulthard [40] suggested that the increased hematocrit following increased dialysis dose is mediated by an increase in endogenous erythropoietin production, rather than enhanced removal of uremic toxins. But in a prospective study of 20 patients in whom hemodialysis dose was increased for 6 weeks percent, an increase in hematocrit was accompanied by a decrease in serum endogenous erythropoietin level – implying that the rise in hematocrit following delivery of good dialysis is not mediated by increased endogenous erythropoietin production [33].

This finding is consistent with other reports showing a decline in endogenous erythropoietin following an increase in hematocrit after blood transfusion, or an increase after acute blood loss or hypoxic stimulus [38,39,41], confirming that the negative feedback that exists in health, is preserved in ESRD. On the other hand, evidence for a possible role for endogenous erythropoietin in erythropoiesis in ESRD is that in patients with ESRD who have autosomal dominant polycystic kidney disease (ADPKD) [42], or viral hepatitis [43,44], anemia is lessened by their increased levels of endogenous erythropoietin.

Dialysis adequacy and RBC lifespan

Whether better dialysis in EPO-treated uremic patients improves anemia via additional mechanisms such as improved red blood cell survival, is unknown. There are conflicting data on whether uremia-induced shortened red blood cell life span improves appreciably with dialysis or erythropoietin therapy [1,45–47]. Also, the suggestion that volume contraction may contribute to the improvement in anemia with better dialysis in EPO-treated patients, is unvalidated.

Clearly, the bulk of laboratory and clinical studies indicate amelioration of anemia in ESRD patients following increased delivered dialysis results predominantly from enhanced extraction of inhibitor(s) of erythropoiesis [21].

However, it is recognized that in addition to erythropoietin, other kinnins such as insulin-like growth factors I and II, growth hormone, colony stimulating factor, and several interleukins play a role in erythropoiesis, and the effect of improved dialysis on these other factors, is unknown.

Responsiveness to EPO in kidney transplant recipients

Even among kidney transplant recipients with chronic allograft dysfunction treated with EPO, response decreased as glomerular filtration declined [48], and very high endogenous erythropoietin levels fail to stimulate erythropoiesis if excretory function is poor [49–51]. Supporting the thesis that enhanced removal of inhibitors from the serum improves erythropoiesis is the finding that despite a nine fold increase in endogenous erythropoietin level, anemia failed to improve – hematocrit only began to rise with restoration of renal function [50].

Furthermore, following a kidney transplant, moderately increased blood levels of endogenous erythropoietin usually induce complete correction of anemia after successful kidney transplantation [49–51]. With good graft function, erythropoiesis is maintained by "normal" serum erythropoietin levels [49–51]. Evidence from these new kidney transplant recipients suggest that slight increases in renal endogenous erythropoietin levels induce erythropoiesis to the same extent as do large doses of exogenous erythropoietin [49–51]. Moreover, in transplant recipients, serum erythropoietin returns to normal as the hematocrit level increases to greater than 32% [50]. Thereafter, the hematocrit continues to increase to normal levels, while serum erythropoietin remains in the normal range. Thus, restoration of renal function, not ambient erythropoietin level is the dominant variable that improves anemia in new kidney transplant recipients.

CONCLUSION

That higher hematocrits in patients with ESRD improves morbidity and mortality is established. However, considering the increased risk of infection and death associated with excess intravenous iron [52], it is indisputable that how we achieve higher hematocrits is also important. It is prudent that the amount of intravenous iron administered to achieve higher hematocrits be appropriate and not excessive. Patients whose low hematocrit is mainly due to inadequate dialysis and/or other identifiable causes who receive unneeded large doses of intravenous iron are unnecessarily exposed to an increased risk of infections and death, thus nullifying the desired favorable effects of higher hematocrit. There is clear and compelling evidence that adequacy of dialysis is an important variable that must be accounted for to maximize correction of anemia in patients with ESRD.

REFERENCES

1. Xia H, Ebben J, Ma JZ, et al. Hematocrit levels and hospitalization risks in hemodialysis patients. J Am Soc Nephrol. 1999;10:1309–16.
2. Ma JZ, Ebben J, Xia H, et al. Hematocrit level and associated mortality in hemodialysis patients. J Am Soc Nephrol. 1999;10:610–19.
3. Eschbach JW, Funk D, Adamson J, Kuhn J, Scribner BH, Finch CA. Erythropoiesis in patients with renal failure undergoing chronic dialysis. N Engl J Med. 1967; 276:653–8.
4. Macdougall IC. Role of uremic toxins in exacerbating anemia in renal failure. Kidney Int. 2001;59:S67–72.
5. Wallner SF, Vautrin RM. Evidence that inhibition of erythropoiesis is important in the anemia of chronic renal failure. J Lab Clin Med. 1981;97:170–8.
6. Markson JL, Rennie JB. The anemia of chronic renal insufficiency. Scottish Med J. 1956;1:320–2.
7. Radtke HW, Rege AB, LaMarche MB, Bartos D, Campbell RA, Fisher JW. Identification of spermine as an inhibitor of erythropoiesis in patients with chronic renal failure. J Clin Invest. 1981;67:1623–9.
8. Essers U, Muller W, Heintz R. Effect of erythropoietin in normal men and in patients with renal insufficiency. Proc Eur Dial Transplant Assoc. 1974;11:398–402.
9. Saito A, Suzuki I, Chung TG, et al. Separation of an inhibitor of erythropoiesis in "middle molecules" from hemodialysate from patients with chronic renal failure. Clin Chem. 1986;32:1938–41.

10. Ortega JA, Malekzadeh MH, Dukes PP, Ma A, Pennisi AV, Fine RN, Shore NA. Exceptionally high serum erythropoietin activity in an anephric patient with severe anemia. Am J Hematol. 1977;2:299–306.

11. Kushner D, Beckman B, Nguyen L, et al. Polyamines in the anemia of end-stage renal disease. Kidney Int. 1991;39:725–32.

12. Delwiche F, Segal GM, Eschbach JW, et al. Hematopoietic inhibitors in chronic renal failure: lack of in vitro specificity. Kidney Int. 1986:29:641–8.

13. McGonigle RJS, Husserl F, Wallin JD, Fisher JW. Hemodialysis and continuous ambulatory peritoneal dialysis effects on erythropoiesis in renal failure. Kidney Int. 1984;25:430–6.

14. Zappacosta AR, Caro J, Erlev A. Normalization of hematocrit in patients with end-stage renal disease on continuous ambulatory peritoneal dialysis. Am J Med. 1982;72:53–7.

15. Urabe A, Chiba S, Kosaka K, et al. Response of uremic bone marrow cells to erythropoietin in vitro. Scand J Haematol. 1976;17:335–40.

16. Santiago GC, Rao TKS, Laird NM. Effect of dialysis therapy on the hematopoietic system: The National Cooperative Dialysis Study. Kidney Int. 1983;23:S95–S100.

17. Geerlings W, Morris RW, Brunner FP, et al. Factors influencing anemia in dialysis patients. A special survey by the EDTA-ERA Registry. Nephrol Dial Transplantation. 1993;8:585–9.

18. Koch KM, Patyna WD, Shaldon S, Werner E. Anemia of the regular hemodialysis patient and its treatment. Nephron. 1974;12:405–19.

19. Yang CS, Chen SW, Chiang CH, et al. Effects of increasing dialysis dose on serum albumin and mortality in hemodialysis patients. Am J Kidney Dis. 1996;27:380–6.

20. Frankenfield D, Johnson CA, Wish JB, Rocco MV, Madore F, Owen WF Jr, for the ESRD Core Indicators Workgroup. Anemia management of adult hemodialysis patients in the U.S.: results from the 1997 ESRD core indicators project. Kidney Int. 2000;57:578–89.

21. Ifudu O, Feldman J, Friedman EA. The intensity of hemodialysis and the response to erythropoietin in patients with end-stage renal disease. N Engl J Med. 1996; 334:420–5.

22. McClellan WM, Frankenfield DL, Wish JB, et al. Subcutaneous erythropoietin results in lower dose and equivalent hematocrit levels among adult hemodialysis patients: results from the 1998 end-stage renal disease core indicators project. Am J Kidney Dis. 2001;37:E36.

23. Madore F, Lowrie E, Brugnara C, et al. Anaemia in hemodialysis patients: variables affecting this outcome predictor. J Am Soc Nephrol. 1997;8:1921–9.

24. Ifudu O, Uribarri J, Rajwani I, Vlacich V, Reydel K, Delosreyes G, Friedman EA. Adequacy of dialysis and differences in hematocrit among dialysis facilities. Am J Kidney Dis. 2000;36:1166–74.

25. National Kidney Foundation-Dialysis Outcomes Quality Initiative (NKF-DOQI) Clinical Practice Guidelines for the Treatment of Anemia of Chronic Renal Failure. Am J Kidney Dis. 1997;30:S192–S237.

26. Health Care Financing Administration. 1998 Annual Report, End Stage Renal Disease Core Indicators Project. Department of Health and Human Services, Health Care Financing Administration, Office of Clinical Standards and Quality, Baltimore, Maryland, December, 1998.

27. Cotter JC, Thamer M, Kimmel PL, et al. Secular trends in recombinant erythropoietin therapy among the U.S. hemodialysis population: 1990–1996. Kidney Int. 1998;54:2129–39.

28. Cohen D, Raja RM. Erythropoietin requirements remain high in erythropoietin resistant patients after iron repletion. ASAIO J. 1998;44:M596–7.

29. Ifudu O, Friedman EA. Economic implications of inadequate response to erythropoietin in patients with end-stage renal disease. Dial Transplantation. 1997;26:664–9.
30. Allen DA, Breen C, Yaqoob MM, Macdougall IC. Inhibition of CFU-E colony formation in uremic patients with inflammatory disease: role of IFN-gamma and TNF-alpha. J Invest Med. 1999;47:204–11.
31. Opatrna S, Opatrny K, Jr, Cejkova' P, et al. Relationship between anemia and adequacy of continuous ambulatory peritoneal dialysis. Nephron. 1997;77:359–60.
32. Tzamaloukas AH, Murata GH, Sena P. When do plasma levels of azotemic indices indicate inadequacy of peritoneal dialysis? Nephron. 1994;67:495–6.
33. Ifudu O, Friedman EA. Effect of increased hemodialysis dose on endogenous erythropoietin production in end-stage renal disease. Nephron. 1998;79:50–4.
34. Movilli E, Cancarini GC, Zani R, Camerini C, et al. Adequacy of dialysis reduces the doses of recombinant erythropoietin independently from the use of biocompatible membranes in haemodialysis patients. Nephrol Dial Transplantation. 2001;16:111–4.
35. Scaini P, Sandrini M, Zani R, et al. Adequacy reduces erythropoietin dose in peritoneal dialysis patients [Abstract]. Nephrol Dial Transplantation. 1999;14:A258.
36. Depner TA, Rizwan S, James LA. Effectiveness of low dose erythropoietin: a possible advantage of high flux hemodialysis. ASAIO Trans. 1990;36:M223–5.
37. Locatelli F, Andrulli S, Pecchini F, Pedrini L, et al. Effect of high-flux dialysis on the anaemia of haemodialysis patients. Nephrol Dial Transplantation. 2000;15:1399–409.
38. Naets JP, Garcia JF, Tousaaint C, Buset M, Waks D. Radioimmunoassay of erythropoietin in chronic uremic or anephric patients. Scand J Haematol. 1986;37:390–4.
39. Kato A, Hishida A, Kumagai H, Furuya R, Nakajima T, Honda N. Erythropoietin production in patients with chronic renal failure. Renal Failure. 1994;16:645–51.
40. Morris K, Coulthard M. End-stage kidneys are capable of increased erythropoietin production. Pediatr Nephrol. 1993;7:273–5.
41. Walle AJ, Wong GY, Clemons GK, Garcia JF, Niedermayer W. Erythropoietin-hematocrit feedback circuit in the anemia of end-stage renal disease. Kidney Int. 1987;31:1205–9.
42. Chandra M, Miller ME, Garcia JF, Mossey RT, McVicar M. Serum immunoreactive erythropoietin levels in patients with polycystic kidney disease as compared with other hemodialysis patients. Nephron. 1985;39:26–9.
43. Ifudu O, Fowler A. Hepatitis B virus infection and the response to erythropoietin in end-stage renal disease. ASAIO J. 2001;47:569–72.
44. Chan N, Barton CH, Mirahmadi MS, et al. Erythropoiesis associated with viral hepatitis in end-stage renal disease. Am J Med Sci. 1984;287:56–8.
45. Shaw AB. Hemolysis in chronic renal failure. Br Med J. 1967;2:213–16.
46. Hartitzsch BV, Carr D, Kjellstrand CM, Kerr DNS. Normal red cell survival in well dialyzed patients. Trans ASAIO. 1973;19:471–4.
47. Najean Y, Moynot A, Deschryver F, Zins B, Naret C, Jacquot C, Drueke T. Kinetics of erythropoiesis in dialysis patients receiving recombinant erythropoietin. Nephrol Dial Transplantation. 1989;4:350–5.
48. Muirhead N, Cattran DC, Zaltzman J, et al. Safety and efficacy of recombinant human erythropoietin in correcting the anemia of patients with chronic renal allograft dysfunction. J Am Soc Nephrol. 1994;5:1216–22.

49. Sun CH, Ward HJ, Paul WL, et al. Serum erythropoietin levels after renal transplantation. N Engl J Med. 1989;321:151–7.
50. Wolff M, Jelkmann W. Erythropoiesis and erythropoietin levels in renal transplant recipients. Klin Wochenschr. 1991;69:53–8.
51. Lee DB. Interrelationship between erythropoietin and erythropoiesis: insights from renal transplantation. Am J Kidney Dis. 1991;18:54–6.
52. Ifudu O. Parenteral iron: pharmacology and clinical use. Nephron. 1998;80: 249–56.

10. Do ACE inhibitors limit response to EPO and should EPO be continued in patients with sepsis or fever?

Moro O. Salifu

INTRODUCTION

Angiotensin-converting-enzyme inhibitors (ACEI) are a class of antihypertensive drugs that block the formation of angiotensin II, thereby abrogating the vasoconstrictive and trophic properties of this compound. They have been shown to decrease cardiovascular mortality [1] and decline in progression of both diabetic and non-diabetic renal disease [2,3]. The cardiovascular benefit of ACEI may be extended to patients with end stage renal disease on dialysis given the high prevalence of diabetes, hypertension and other risk factors [4,5]. Among other side effects such as cough and hyperkalemia, one observation of interest is the development or worsening of anemia and increased requirement for erythropoietin (EPO) when ACEI are used in dialysis or transplant patients. It has been suggested that ACEI may induce anemia in dialysis patients by reducing the production of residual endogenous EPO, by raising serum levels of an inhibitor of erythropoiesis or directly inhibiting bone marrow erythropoiesis. Clinical studies, mostly retrospective data addressing this question have been anecdotal. While some studies suggest that anemia can be induced by ACEI in dialysis patients, others do not support this notion. The controversy regarding the use of EPO in dialysis patients with fever or sepsis will also be discussed.

Overview of EPO physiology

Erythropoietin is a glycoprotein primarily produced in the outer medulla and cortex of the kidney by peritubular fibroblast-like type 1 interstitial cells [6–8]. EPO is produced in response to tissue hypoxia induced by

Onyekachi Ifudu (ed.), Renal Anemia: Conflicts and Controversies, 99–106.
© 2002 Kluwer Academic Publishers.

hypoxemia, anemia, volume depletion, catecholamines and angiotensin II. Adenosine [9], produced as a result of tissue hypoxia is thought to be an intermediary molecule stimulating the oxygen sensor located on cell membranes of these cells to produce EPO. Thus adenosine antagonists [10,11] have been used for the treatment of posttransplant erythrocytosis. Angiotensin II and catcholamines induce EPO production via renal afferent arteriolar vasoconstriction thereby leading to decreased oxygen delivery but increased oxygen consumption because of increased proximal tubular reabsorption of sodium [12]. EPO secreted from these mechanisms gets to the bone marrow via circulation where it is required for the maturation of erythroid cell lines [13] particularly the conversion of burst forming units (BFU) to colony forming units (CFU) and from CFU to proerythroblast.

Relationship between the renin angiotensin system and erythropoiesis

The stimulation of EPO production by the renin angiotensin system in chronic dialysis patients has been demonstrated in several studies. Vlahakos et al. [12] showed that patients on chronic hemodialysis not requiring exogenous EPO but maintaining mean hematocrit of 32% had significantly higher mean plasma renin activity than those on exogenous erythropoietin with similar hematocrit and blood pressure. Volume depletion in the group not on EPO was associated with an increase in PRA with concomitant increase in serum EPO levels. The increase in EPO with volume depletion was abolished when captopril was given before volume depletion suggesting that EPO production was mediated in part by the renin angiotensin system. This association may explain why use of converting enzyme inhibitors in dialysis patients has been associated with anemia or higher requirements for EPO [14] and a decrease in hematocrit when patients with posttransplant erythrocytosis are treated with converting enzyme inhibitors [15–17] or angiotensin II receptor blocker [18].

   In addition to stimulation of EPO production through renal vasoconstriction, angiotensin II induces proliferation of bone marrow progenitor cells [19,20] from murine or human cord blood. Murine or human progenitor cells incubated with different concentrations of angiotensin II for up to two weeks demonstrate a concentration dependent increase in colony formation. Angiotensin II-induced colony formation is inhibited by addition of losartan, an angiotensin II receptor antagonist [20], suggesting the presence of angiotensin II receptors on these cell lines. In this study, angiotensin II receptors were identified in different bone marrow cell lines except granulocytes. Angiotensin II receptor blockade (losartan 50 mg/d) has been used successfully to treat posttransplant polycythemia in renal transplant recipients [18].

Another relationship between RAS and erythropoiesis is the regulation of a natural stem cell regulator found in circulation called AcSDKP (N-acetyl-seryl-aspartyl-lysyl-proline [21]. Ac-SDKP is a potent reversible inhibitor of stem cell proliferation by preventing stem cells from entering S-phase of the cell cycle [22]. AcSDKP is deactivated by hydrolysis by angiotensin converting enzyme [23]. Inhibition of angiotensin converting enzyme would therefore result in elevation of plasma Ac-SDKP levels, inhibition of stem cell proliferation and erythropoiesis [24]. In 8 healthy volunteers, a single 50 mg dose of captopril, an angiotensin converting enzyme inhibitor, resulted in a 5-fold increase in plasma levels of AcSDKP when compared to placebo and also induced 90–99% inhibition of invitro hydrolysis of AcSDKP [25]. ACEI therapy has been associated with reduced IGF-1 [26] and IL-12 [27] serum levels, both of which are stimulators of erythropoiesis.

From the foregoing, it is apparent that there is no unifying mechanism for the inhibition of erythropoiesis by ACEI. The combination of several mechanisms can be summarized as decreased EPO production, direct bone marrow suppression and increased circulating levels of the stem cell inhibitor Ac-SDKP.

Evidence for ACEI-induced anemia

These studies suggest that there is an effect of ACEI on hemoglobin or hematocrit and increased requirement for EPO in EPO-treated patients. In a retrospective study of 43 patients (20 on captopril, 23 controls), Walter et al. [28], showed that captopril treated patients had significantly lower hemoglobin in the captopril-treated patients (6.2 ± 0.2 vs. 7.1 ± 0.2 g/dl, $p < 0.0$). In a similar retrospective study Erturk et al. [29] showed that patients on ACEI ($n = 47$, 23 on ACEI, 24 control) had mean lower hematocrit than those not on ACEI ($25.8 \pm 6.4\%$ vs. $32.0 \pm 4.2\%$, $p < 0.001$). EPO requirement was higher in the ACEI treated group. Matsumura et al. [30] found that EPO requirement were higher in ACEI-treated patients in a retrospective study of 108 patients (49 on ACEI, 49 controls). In a prospective study of 60 patients (20 on enalapril, 20 on nifedipine and 20 controls) followed up to 12 months, Albitar et al. [31] found that patients on enalapril required higher doses EPO than nifedipine or controls. Similarly, Hess et al. [32] found higher requirement for EPO in ACEI-treated patients. In a small prospective uncontrolled study of 15 patients, withdrawal of ACEI in patents on EPO caused an increase in hematocrit and decrease in EPO dose [33]. ACEI-induced anemia or increase in EPO requirement have been found in other studies [34,35] as well as in patients on peritoneal dialysis [36,37].

Evidence against ACEI-induced anemia

These studies suggest that there is no effect of ACEI on hemoglobin or hematocrit in EPO-treated patients. In 14 hemodialysis patients studied retrospectively, Colon et al. [38] found no difference in mean hematocrit before and after starting ACEI. In 252 patients (48 on ACEI, 204 controls) studied retrospectively, Sanchez et al. [39] found no difference in hemoglobin, hematocrit or EPO dose in EPO-treated vs. controls. Similarly, in a retrospective study of 48 (24 ACEI, 24 control) Cruz et al. [40], found no difference in hematocrit or EPO in EPO-treated vs. controls. In yet another retrospective study of 175 (32 on ACEI, 143 control) patients receiving chronic dialysis treated with EPO for at least 3 months, Charytan et al. [41] found that neither dose nor duration of ACEI therapy affected the response to EPO. Schwenk et al. also found no difference in EPO requirement in ACEI treated patient vs. controls [42]. The angiotensin II receptor blocker, losartan did not have any effect on response to erythropoietin therapy in patients undergoing hemodialysis [43,44].

CONCLUSION

Given the available evidence, there is insufficient evidence to preclude the use of ACEI or angiotensin II receptor blockers in dialysis patients. The cardiovascular benefit of ACEI in these high-risk populations therefore outweighs the potential decrease in hemoglobin or hematocrit values, an effect, which can be offset by increasing the dose of EPO.

Recommendation

Other causes of anemia or EPO resistance [45] must be vigorously sought and corrected. The indication for ACEI therapy in an individual patient should be reassessed routinely if target hemoglobin of 11–12 g/dl is not achieved, despite > 200 U/kg/week of EPO [46]. Under these circumstances, if no other cause for EPO resistance is identified, a trial of reducing the dose of ACEI (if absolutely indicated such as heart failure) or switching to another antihypertensive drug may be prudent.

Should EPO be used in patients with fever or sepsis

Acute or chronic inflammation with or without infection results in a state of significant EPO resistance because of impaired release and utilization of iron (reticulo-endothelial block), the inhibition of erythropoiesis by circulating inflammatory cytokines such as TNF-α, IL-1, IFN-γ [47–49], decreased endogenous EPO synthesis [50,51] and decreased red blood cell survival [52]. There are no studies to support continuation or discontinuation of EPO during fever or sepsis. Based on the available evidence above, it is prudent to suggest doubling of the EPO dose and switching from the intravenous to subcutaneous routes [53] if the EPO response is not met. It is unlikely that additional benefit of increasing the EPO dose will be achieved without vigorously searching for and treating the cause of fever or sepsis.

REFERENCES

1. Yusuf S, Sleight P, Pogue J, Bosch J, Davies R, Dagenais G. Effects of an angiotensin-converting-enzyme inhibitor, ramipril, on cardiovascular events in high-risk patients. The Heart Outcomes Prevention Evaluation Study Investigators. N Engl J Med. 2000;342:145–53.
2. Lewis EJ, Hunsicker LG, Bain RP, Rohde RD. The effect of angiotensin-converting-enzyme inhibition on diabetic nephropathy. The Collaborative Study Group. N Engl J Med. 1993;329:1456–62.
3. Ruggenenti P, Perna A, Gherardi G, Garini G, Zoccali C, Salvadori M, Scolari F, Schena FP, Remuzzi G. Renoprotective properties of ACE-inhibition in non-diabetic nephropathies with non-nephrotic proteinuria. Lancet. 1999;354:359–64.
4. Collins AJ, Li S, Ma JZ, Herzog C. Cardiovascular disease in end-stage renal disease patients. Am J Kidney Dis. 2001;38:S26–9.
5. U.S. Renal Data System: USRDS 2000 Annual Data Report, The National Institute of Health, National Institute of Diabetes and Digestive and Kidney Diseases, Bethesda, MD, June 2000.
6. Kurtz A, Eckardt KU, Neumann R, Kaissling B, LeHir M, Bauer C. Site of erythropoietin formation. Contr Nephrol. 1989;76:14–23.
7. Koury ST, Bondurant MC, Koury MJ. Localization of erythropoietin sensitizing cells in murine kidney by in situ hybridization. Blood. 1988;71:524–7.
8. Lacombe C, Da Silva JL, Bruneval P, Fournier JG, Wendling F, Casadevall N, Camilleri JP, Bariety J, Varet B, Tambourin P. Peritubular cells are the site of erythropoietin synthesis in the murine hypoxic kidney. J Clin Invest. 1988;81:620–3.
9. Scholz H, Schurek HJ, Eckardt KU, Bauer C. Role of erythropoietin in adaptation to hypoxia. Experientia. 1990;46:1197–201.
10. Osswald H, Gleiter C, Muhlbauer B. Therapeutic use of theophylline to antagonize renal effects of adenosine. Clin Nephrol. 1995;43(supplement 1):S33–7.
11. Grekas D, Dioudis C, Valkouma D, Papoulidou F, Tourkantonis A. Theophylline modulates erythrocytosis after renal transplantation. Nephron. 1995;70:25–7.

12. Vlahakos DV, Balodimos C, Papachristopoulos V, Vassilakos P, Hinari E, Vlacho-jannis JG. Renin angiotensin system stimulates erythropoietin secretion in chronic hemodialysis patients. Clin Nephrol. 1995;43:53–59.

13. Freyssinier JM, Lecoq-Lafon C, Amsellem S, Picard F, Ducrocq R, Mayeux P, Lacombe C, Fichelson S. Purification, amplification and characterization of a population of human erythroid progenitors. Br J Haematol. 1999;106:912–22.

14. Hess E, Sperschneider H, Stein G. Do ACE inhibitors influence the dose of human recombinant erythropoietin in dialysis patients? Nephrol Dial Transplantation. 1996;11:749–51.

15. Vlahakos DV, Canzanello VJ, Madaio MP, Madias NE. Enalapril-associated anemia in renal transplant recipients treated for hypertension. Am J Kidney Dis. 1991; 17:199–205.

16. Perazella M, McPherdran P, Kliger A, Lorber M, Levy E, Bia MJ. Enalapril treatment of Posttransplant Erythrocytosis: Am J Kidney Dis. 1995;26:495–500.

17. Suh BY, Suh JD, Kwun KB. Effect of caporal in the treatment of erythrocytosis after renal transplantation. Transpl Proc. 1996;28:1557–8.

18. Kupin W, Venkat KK, Goggins M et al. Benefit of angiotensin II receptor blockade in the treatment of posttransplant polycytemia in renal transplant recipients. Transpl Proc. 1997;29:207–8.

19. Mrug M, Stopka T, Julian BA, Prchal JF, Prchal JT. Angiotensin II stimulates proliferation of normal early erythroid progenitors. J Clin Invest. 1997;100: 2310–4.

20. Rodgers KE, Xiong S, Steer R, diZerega GS. Effect of angiotensin II on hematopoietic progenitor cell proliferation. Stem Cells. 2000;18:287–94.

21. Lenfant M, Wdzieczak-Bakala J, Guittet E, Prome JC, Sotty D and Frindel E. Inhibitor of hematopoietic pluripotent stem cell proliferation: purification and determination of its structure. Proc Natl Acad Sci USA. 1989;86: 779–82.

22. Bonnet D, Lemoine FM, Ponvert-Delucq S, Baillou C, Najman A, Guignon M. Direct and reversible inhibitory effect of the tetrapeptide acetyl-N-ser-asp-lys-pro (serapenide) on the growth of human CD34+ subpopulations in response to growth factors. Blood. 1993;82:3307–14.

23. Rieger K-J, Saez-Servent N, Papet M-P, Wdzieczak-Bakala J, Morgat J-L, Thierry J, Voelter W, Lenfant M. Involvement of human plasma angiotensin I-converting enzyme in the degradation of the haemoregulatory peptide N-acetyl seryl aspartyl lysyl proline. Biochem J. 1993; 296:1–6.

24. Le Meur Y, Lorgeot V, Comte L, Szelag JC, Aldigier JC, Leroux-Robert C, Praloran V. Plasma levels and metabolism of AcSDKP in patients with chronic renal failure: relationship with erythropoietin requirements. Am J Kidney Dis. 2001; 38:510–17.

25. Azizi M, Rousseau A, Ezan E, Guyene T, Michelet S, Grognet J, Lenfant M, Corvol P, Ménard J. Acute angiotensin-converting enzyme inhibition increases the plasma level of the natural stem cell regulator N-acetyl-seryl-aspartyl-lysyl-proline. J Clin Invest. 1996;97:839–44.

26. Morrone LF, Di Paolo S, Logoluso F, Schena A, Stallone G, Giorgino F, Schena FP. Interference of angiotensin-converting enzyme inhibitors on erythropoiesis in kidney transplant recipients: role of growth factors and cytokines. Transplanta-tion. 1997;64:913–8.

27. Constantinescu CS, Goodman DB, Ventura ES. Captopril and lisinopril suppress production of interleukin-12 by human peripheral blood mononuclear cells. Immunol Lett. 1998;62:25–31.

28. Walter J. Does captopril decrease the effect of human recombinant erythropoietin in hemodialysis patients? Nephrol Dial Transplantation. 1993;8:1428.

29. Erturk S, Ates K, Duman N, Karatan O, Erbay B, Ertug E. Unresponsiveness to recombinant human erythropoietin in haemodialysis patients: possible implications of angiotensin converting enzyme inhibitors. Nephrol Dial Transplantation. 1996;11:396–97.
30. Matsumura M, Nomura H, Koni I, Mabuchi H. Angiotensin-converting enzyme inhibitors are associated with the need for increased recombinant human erythropoietin maintenance doses in hemodialysis patients. Nephron. 1997;77:164–8.
31. Albitar S, Genin R, Fen-Chong M, Serveaux M-O, Bourgeon B. High dose enalapril impairs the response to erythropoietin treatment in haemodialysis patients. Nephrol Dial Transplantation. 1998;13:1206–10.
32. Hess E, Sperschneider H, Stein G. Do ACE inhibitors influence the dose of human recombinant erythropoietin in dialysis patients? Nephrol Dial Transplantation. 1996;11:749–51.
33. Erturk S, Nergizoglu G, Ates K, Duman N, Erbay B, Karatan O, Ertug AE. The impact of weaning of ACE inhibitors on erythropoietin responsiveness and left ventricular hypertrophy in haemodialysis patients. Nephrol Dial Transplantation. 1999;14:1912–16.
34. Onoyama K, Sanai T, Motomura K, Fujishima M. Worsening of anemia by angiotensin converting enzyme inhibitors and its prevention by antiestrogenic steroid in chronic hemodialysis patients. J Cardiovasc Pharmacol. 1989;13:S27–30.
35. Dhondt AW, Vanholder RC, Ringoir SM. Angiotensin-converting enzyme inhibitors and higher erythropoietin requirement in chronic haemodialysis patients. Nephrol Dial Transplantation. 1995;10:2107–9.
36. Mora C, Navarro JF. Negative effect of angiotensin-converting enzyme inhibitors on erythropoietin response in CAPD patients. Am J Nephrol. 2000;20:248.
37. Navarro JF, Macia ML, Mora-Fernandez C, Gallego E, Chahin J, Mendez ML, del Castillo N, Rivero A, Garcia J. Effects of angiotensin-converting enzyme inhibitors on anemia and erythropoietin requirements in peritoneal dialysis patients. Adv Peritoneal Dial. 1997;13:257-9.
38. Conlon PJ, Albers F, Butterly D, Schwab SJ. ACE inhibitors do not affect erythropoietin efficacy in haemodialysis patients. Nephrol Dial Transplantation. 1994;9:1358.
39. Sánchez JA. ACE inhibitors do not decrease r-HuEPO response in patients with end-stage renal failure. Nephrol Dial Transplantation. 1995;10:1476–7.
40. Cruz DN, Perazella MA, Abu-Alfa AK, Mahnensmith RL. Angiotensin-converting enzyme inhibitor therapy in chronic hemodialysis patients: any evidence of erythropoietin resistance? Am J Kidney Dis. 1996;28:535–40.
41. Charytan C, Goldfarb-Rumyantzev A, Wang YF, Schwenk MH, Spinowitz BS. Effect of angiotensin-converting enzyme inhibitors on response to erythropoietin therapy in chronic dialysis patients. Am J Nephrol. 1998;18:498–503.
42. Schwenk MH, Jumani AQ, Rosenberg CR, Kulogowski JE, Charytan C, Spinowitz BS. Potential angiotensin-converting enzyme inhibitor-epoetin alfa interaction in patients receiving chronic hemodialysis. Pharmacotherapy. 1998;18:627-30.
43. Kato A, Takita T, Furuhashi M, Takahashi T, Maruyama Y, Hishida A. No effect of losartan on response to erythropoietin therapy in patients undergoing hemodialysis. Nephron. 2000;86:538-9.
44. Chew CG, Weise MD, Disney APS. The effect of angiotensin II receptor antagonist on the exogenous erythropoietin requirement of haemodialysis patients. Nephrol Dial Transplantation. 1999;14:2047–9.
45. Macdougall IC. Poor response to erythropoietin: practical guidelines on investigation and management. Nephrol Dial Transplantation. 1995;10: 607–14.

46. Macdougall IC. The role of ACE inhibitors and angiotensin II receptor blockers in the response to epoetin Nephrol Dial Transplantation. 1999;14:1836–41.
47. Rusten LS, Jacobsen SE. Tumor necrosis factor (TNF)-alpha directly inhibits human erythropoiesis in vitro: role of p55 and p75 TNF receptors. Blood. 1995; 85:989–96.
48. Schooley JC, Kullgren B, Allison AC. Inhibition by interleukin-1 of the action of erythropoietin on erythroid precursors and its possible role in the pathogenesis of hypoplastic anaemias. Br J Haematol. 1987;67:11–17.
49. Allen DA, Breen C, Yaqoob MM, Macdougall IC. Inhibition of CFU-E colony formation in uremic patients with inflammatory disease: role of IFN-gamma and TNF-alpha. J Investig Med. 1999;47:204–11.
50. Rogiers P, Zhang H, Leeman M, Nagler J, Neels H, Melot C, Vincent JL. Erythropoietin response is blunted in critically ill patients. Intensive Care Med. 1997;23:159–62.
51. Abel J, Spannbrucker N, Fandrey J, Jelkmann W. Serum erythropoietin levels in patients with sepsis and septic shock. Eur J Haematol. 1996;57:359–63.
52. Karle H. The pathogenesis of the anaemia of chronic disorders and the role of fever in erythrokinetics. Scand J Haematol. 1974;13:81–6.
53. Besarab A. Physiological and pharmacodynamic considerations for route of EPO administration. Semin Nephrol. 2000;20:364–74.

11. Is secondary hyperparathyroidism a significant cause of renal anemia?

Onyekachi Ifudu

INTRODUCTION

Anemia, a major feature of end-stage renal disease (ESRD) is chiefly due to diminished erythropoietin synthesis by diseased kidneys [1]. It is suggested that parathyroid hormone, when in excessive amounts, interferes with normal erythropoiesis by down regulating the erythropoietin receptors on erythroid progenitor cells in the bone marrow [2]. Therefore, physiologic concentrations of erythropoietin can no longer sustain normal red cell counts, so normocytic and normochromic anemia ensues [2]. In primary hyperparathyroidism, this effect is observed with very high concentrations of parathyroid hormone. In secondary hyperparathyroidism during chronic renal failure, this effect is more pronounced because erythropoietin synthesis is impaired [2].

Anemia (hematocrit ⩽ 30%) persists in as many as 30% of maintenance hemodialysis patients despite recombinant erythropoietin (EPO) therapy. Bone marrow fibrosis associated with secondary hyperparathyroidism would explain – in part – a suboptimal response to EPO therapy in some ESRD patients [3–14]. However, since bone marrow biopsy is an invasive procedure, its application should be selective. Several single-center and uncontrolled studies implicate secondary hyperparathyroidism as a cause for impaired response to EPO therapy. This review weighs the laboratory and clinical evidence supporting a clear relation between secondary hyperparathyroidism and uremic anemia, before and after the emergence of EPO.

Onyekachi Ifudu (ed.), Renal Anemia: Conflicts and Controversies, 107–113.
© 2002 *Kluwer Academic Publishers.*

Anemia in hyperparathyroidism – potential mechanisms

It is postulated that excess parathyroid hormone, impairs erythropoiesis by down regulating the erythropoietin receptors on erythroid progenitor cells in the bone marrow. Thus, physiologic concentrations of erythropoietin can no longer sustain normal red cell production. Investigators have also theorized a direct toxic effect on the red blood cell leading to enhanced hemolysis. In patients with kidney failure, bone marrow fibrosis due to secondary hyperparathyroidism is associated with anemia and suboptimal response to erythropoietin partly because of replacement of the cellular components of the bone marrow by fibrous tissue.

Is parathyroid hormone toxic to RBCs and erythroid progenitors?

In primary hyperparathyroidism, anemia has been observed with very high concentrations of PTH [15,16]. It is postulated that in addition to shortening the red blood cell life span by enhanced hemolysis, elevated PTH level may impair erythropoietin synthesis or induces bone marrow resistance, therefore, physiologic concentrations of erythropoietin can no longer sustain normal erythropoiesis [2,4,17].

Laboratory studies show that parathyroid hormone inhibits growth of erythroid progenitor cells and heme synthesis [6,18]. Meytes et al. [6], reported that in the presence of erythropoietin concentrations equivalent to that found in ESRD patients, parathyroid hormone inhibited growth of mouse bone marrow erythroid burst-forming units (BFU-E) but not that of the mouse erythroid colony-forming units (CFU-E). The authors did not offer an explanation for this disparity in specific cells inhibited by parathyroid hormone, and also found that the inhibition was overcome by addition of EPO [6].

While several investigators have demonstrated a dose-dependent inhibition of erythroid progenitor cells with decreased heme synthesis, these findings have been disputed by investigators who showed that very high parathyroid hormone levels failed to inhibit heme synthesis in *in vitro* cell cultures [19,20].

Also, it is reported that high levels of parathyroid hormone in uremia shortens the life span of red blood cell by elevating their osmotic fragility, inhibits endogenous erythropoietin production, and also limit responsiveness of erythroid progenitor cells to erythropoietin [4-6]. However, it has been shown that serum parathyroid hormone level does not correlate with hematocrit or dose of EPO [3,21].

Marrow fibrosis and anemia

Bone marrow fibrosis due to secondary hyperparathyroidism is associated with anemia and suboptimal response to EPO partly because of replacement of the cellular components (red marrow and erythroid progenitors) of the bone marrow by fibrous tissue [3].

In a study of 18 hemodialysis patients in whom bone histomorphometry was performed, Rao et al. [3], found that percentages of osteoid volume and surface, osteoid thickness were similar in patients who responded well to erythropoietin as well as those with erythropoietin hyporesponse. However the patients with EPO hyporesponse had higher parathyroid hormone levels and greater marrow fibrosis than their counterparts [3]. These authors concluded that responsiveness to EPO was proportional to extent of marrow fibrosis. However, in a study to evaluate the effect of parathyroidectomy on anemia in dialysis patients, Mandolfo et al. [22], did not observe a correlation between degrees of marrow fibrosis and anemia before parathyroidectomy nor between degree of fibrosis and improvement of anemia after parathyroidectomy.

Of the known causes of EPO hyporesponse in ESRD patients, bone marrow fibrosis associated with secondary hyperparathyroidism is the most difficult to document, because it entails performance of bone marrow biopsy – an invasive and painful procedure [3]. In clinical practice, bone marrow biopsy is often a last resort in the evaluation of persistent anemia.

Effect of parathyroidectomy on anemia

In primary hyperparathyroidism, surgical ablation of parathyroid adenoma has been shown to correct anemia [15,16]. However, there are conflicting data dating back to the preEPO era, on whether anemia improves after parathyroidectomy in ESRD patients with secondary hyperparathyroidism [5,13,22–27]. While some single-center and uncontrolled studies found improved anemia or reduced EPO requirment after parathyroidectomy, other investigators did not. Moreover, even in the positive studies, often, majority of the study subjects did not evince any improvement in anemia after parathyroidectomy. For example, in the study by Podjarny et al. [25], in the preEPO era (1981), anemia improved in only 44% of their ESRD patients after parathyroidectomy. Furthermore, investigators have failed to consistently demonstrate improved responsiveness to EPO or reduced EPO requirement following parathyroidectomy in persons with ESRD.

The failure to obtain a consistent outcome with regard to anemia severity or EPO requirement after parathyroidectomy in patients with obvious secondary hyperparathyroidism is unexplained. Is it possible that after a certain point, severe and prolonged marrow fibrosis may become irreversible and erythropoiesis may remain permanently impaired? However, it is worth noting that there is no correlation between hematocrit level and biochemical indices of secondary hyperparathyroidism [25]. This is consistent with findings that serum parathyroid hormone level does not correlate with neither hematocrit no EPO dose in ESRD patients [3,21].

That bone marrow fibrosis associated with secondary hyperparathyroidism, is associated with relative resistance to EPO therapy is undisputed [3]. However, because bone marrow is invasive and painful, performance of bone marrow biopsy to diagnose marrow fibrosis is often a last resort in the evaluation of persistent anemia. The challenge is coming up with a set of predictors to ascertain who has the high likely hood of having marrow fibrosis, thus the need for biopsy. Because if parathyroidectomy is going to be preformed because of persistent anemia and EPO hyporesponse, then marrow fibrosis should be documented.

Otherwise hemodialysis patients with undiagnosed marrow fibrosis, may continue to receive large inefficacious doses of EPO, at a considerable cost to the system, with increased potential for side effects. Thus, it will be helpful if we can predict those with an increased risk of bone marrow fibrosis.

In a prospective study of 35 randomly selected EPO-treated hemodialysis patients to determine whether their serum levels of intact parathyroid hormone might serve as a marker to detect those who respond poorly to EPO therapy, it was found that serum intact parathyroid hormone did not have a significant correlation with hematocrit ($r = 0.026$; $p = 0.88$). Also, regression analysis with adjustment for EPO dose showed that serum intact parathyroid hormone ($p = 0.12$) did not have a statistically significant relationship with the hematocrit. [21]. The authors concluded that serum levels of intact parathyroid hormone does not detect poor responders to EPO therapy in patients with ESRD [21].

Effect of medical treatment of secondary hyperparathyroidism on anemia

In ESRD patients with severe secondary hyperparathyroidism and anemia treatment with active vitamin D analogues have been shown to result in improved anemia as well as reduction in EPO requirement [10,28]. In these single center and uncontrolled studies, the investigators found that amelioration of anemia was accompanied with concomitant decline in intact serum parathyroid hormone level.

CONCLUSION

A pathogenetic role of secondary hyperparathyroidism in the anemia of chronic renal failure has clearly been demonstrated. However, based on available data, the relative contribution of secondary hyperparathyroidism to uremic anemia remains unclear. While there is compelling data that marrow fibrosis induced by secondary hyperparathyroidism induces anemia and poor response to erythropoietin, available data suggest that the magnitude of a direct effect of excess parathyroid hormone on red blood cells and/or erythroid progenitor cells in uremia, is probably small.

Though there are several reasons justifying parathyroidectomy in ESRD patients with osteodystrophy, marrow fibrosis should be confirmed if anemia is the major impetus for elective parathyroidectomy. The quagmire is that serum parathyroid hormone does not correlate with neither hemartocrit nor erythropoietin dose.

A key research question that needs to be addressed is to define markers to identify those poor responders to erythropoietin during maintenance hemodialysis who should receive a bone marrow biopsy to confirm marrow fibrosis, after excluding all other easily identifiable causes. This is pertinent, since many hemodialysis patients with undiagnosed bone marrow fibrosis, may continue to receive large doses of erythropoietin for prolonged periods, resulting in wasteful administration of an expensive drug, with added potential for side effects. Also, studies are needed to determine why anemia fails to ameliorate in some patients with marrow fibrosis due secondary hyperparathyroidism following parathyroidectomy.

REFERENCES

1. Eschbach JW. The anemia of chronic renal failure: pathophysiology and the effects of recombinant erythropoietin. Kidney Int. 1989;35:134–48.
2. Sikole A. Pathogenesis of anaemia in hyperparathyroidism. Med Hypotheses. 2000;54:236–8.
3. Rao SD, Shih M, Mohini R. Effect of serum parathyroid hormone and bone marrow fibrosis on the response to erythropoietin in uremia. N Engl J Med. 1993; 328:171–5.
4. Malachi T, Bogin E, Gafter U, Levi J. Parathyroid hormone effect on the fragility of human young and old red blood cells in uremia. Nephron. 1986;42:52–7.

5. Urena P, Eckhardt KU, Sarfati E, Zingraff J, Zins B, Roullet JB, Roland E, Drueke T, Kurtz A. Serum erythropoietin and erythropoiesis in primary and secondary hyperparathyroidism: effects of parathyroidectomy. Nephron. 1991;59:384–93.

6. Meytes D, Bogin E, Ma A, Dukes PP, Massry SG. Effect of parathyroid hormone on erythropoiesis. J Clin Invest. 1981;67:1263–9.

7. Seeherunvong W, Rubio L, Abitbol CL, Montane B, Strauss J, Diaz R, Zilleruelo G. Identification of poor responders to erythropoietin among children undergoing hemodialysis. J Pediatr. 2001;138:710–4.

8. Macdougall IC. Role of uremic toxins in exacerbating anemia in renal failure. Kidney Int. 2001;78:S67–72.

9. Kcomt J, Sotelo C, Raja R. Influence of adynamic bone disease on responsiveness to recombinant human erythropoietin in peritoneal dialysis patients. Adv Peritoneal Dial. 2000;16:294–6.

10. Goicoechea M, Vazquez MI, Ruiz MA, Gomez-Campdera F, Perez-Garcia R, Valderrabano F. Intravenous calcitriol improves anaemia and reduces the need for erythropoietin in haemodialysis patients. Nephron. 1998;78:23–7.

11. Belsha CW, Berry PL. Effect of hyperparathyroidism on response to erythropoietin in children on dialysis. Pediatr Nephrol. 1998;12:298–303.

12. Fujita Y, Inoue S, Horiguchi S, Kuki A. Excessive level of parathyroid hormone may induce the reduction of recombinant human erythropoietin effect on renal anemia. Miner Electrolyte Metab. 1995;21:50–4.

13. Goicoechea M, Gomez-Campdera F, Polo JR, Tejedor A, Ruiz MA, Vazquez I, Verde E, Valderrabano F. Secondary hyperparathyroidism as cause of resistance to treatment with erythropoietin: effect of parathyroidectomy. Clin Nephrol 1996; 45:420–1.

14. McGonigle RJ, Wallin JD, Husserl F, Deftos LJ, Rice JC, O'Neill WJ Jr, Fisher JW. Potential role of parathyroid hormone as an inhibitor of erythropoiesis in the anemia of renal failure. J Lab Clin Med. 1984;104(6):1016–26.

15. Falko JM, Guy JT, Smith RE, Mazzaferri EL. Primary hyperparathyroidism and anemia. Arch Intern Med. 1976;136(8):887–9.

16. Boxer M, Ellman L, Geller R, Wang CA. Anemia in primary hyperparathyroidism. Arch Intern Med. 1977;137(5):588–93.

17. Bogin E, Massry SG, Levi J, Djaldeti M, Bristol G, Smith J. Effect of parathyroid hormone on osmotic fragility of human erythrocytes. J Clin Invest. 1982;69(4): 1017–25.

18. Dunn CD, Trent D. The effect of parathyroid hormone on erythropoiesis in serum-free cultures of fetal mouse liver cells. Proc Soc Exp Biol Med. 1981;166(4):556–61.

19. Delwiche F, Garrity MJ, Powell JS, Robertson RP, Adamson JW. High levels of the circulating form of parathyroid hormone do not inhibit in vitro erythropoiesis. J Lab Clin Med. 1983;102(4):613–20.

20. Komatsuda A, Hirokawa M, Haseyama T, Horiuchi T, Wakui H, Imai H, Miura AB. Human parathyroid hormone does not influence human erythropoiesis in vitro. Nephrol Dial Transplantation. 1998;13(8):2088–91.

21. Ifudu O, Homel P. Effect of serum parathyroid hormone and aluminum levels on the response to erythropoietin in uremia. Nephron. 1998;79:477–8.

22. Mandolfo S, Malberti F, Farina M, Villa G, Scanziani R, Surian M, Imbasciati E. Parathyroidectomy and response to erythropoietin therapy in anaemic patients with chronic renal failure. Nephrol Dial Transplantation. 1998;13(10):2708–9.

23. Coen G, Calabria S, Bellinghieri G, Pecchini F, Conte F, Chiappini MG, Ferrannini M, Lagona C, Mallamace A, Manni M, DiLuca M, Sardella D, Taggi F. Parathyroidectomy in chronic renal failure: short- and long-term results on parathyroid function, blood pressure and anemia. Nephron. 2001;88:149–55.

24. Washio M, Iseki K, Onoyama K, Oh Y, Nakamoto M, Fujimi S, Fujishima M. Elevation of serum erythropoietin after subtotal parathyroidectomy in chronic haemodialysis patients. Nephrol Dial Transplantation. 1992;7(2):121–4.

25. Podjarny E, Rathaus M, Korzets Z, Blum M, Zevin D, Bernheim J. Is anemia of chronic renal failure related to secondary hyperparathyroidism? Arch Intern Med. 1981;141(4):453–5.

26. Barbour GL. Effect of parathyroidectomy on anemia in chronic renal failure. Arch Intern Med. 1979;139(8):889–91.

27. Rault R, Magnone M. The effect of parathyroidectomy on hematocrit and erythropoietin dose in patients on hemodialysis. ASAIO J. 1996;42(5):M901–3.

28. Argiles A, Lorho R, Mourad G, Mion CM. High-dose alfacalcidol for anaemia in dialysis. Lancet. 1993;342(8867):378–9.

12. Is long-term intravenous iron therapy risky?

Wendy L. St. Peter

INTRODUCTION

Iron overload was a common problem in patients with chronic kidney disease (CKD) treated with dialysis before the availability of recombinant human erythropoietin (rHuEPO). Iron overload during that time was mainly due to a combination of a hypoproliferative erythroid bone marrow along with frequent administration of packed red blood cell (PRBC) transfusions to manage symptomatic anemia [1]. The result of iron overload was hepatomegaly, hypersplenism and hyperpigmentation. Cirrhosis could also develop as a result of transfusion-related hepatitis infection. Intravenous (IV) iron has also been reported to cause iron overload in patients concomitantly receiving PRBCs in the pre-rHuEPO era [1]. The use of IV iron with or without concomitant PRBCs also contributed to iron overloading in the past and was associated with iron deposits in liver reticuloendothelial and parenchymal cells. However, iron overloading was not associated with functional changes in the liver (i.e., increases in liver function tests or cirrhosis) unless PRBC transfusions resulted in viral hepatitis [1].

The availability of rHuEPO has eliminated the need for routine administration of PRBCs to maintain hematocrit. Stimulating erythropoiesis with rHuEPO also has the added benefit of mobilizing stored iron for incorporation into newly synthesized hemoglobin. In fact, an era of iron overload has now transitioned to an era of relative iron deficiency. Adequate iron stores are critical to achieve an optimal response to rHuEPO. Oral iron has been found to be inadequate to replete and maintain iron supplies in hemodialysis patients, thus, IV iron has become a mainstay in the treatment of anemia in this patient population [2]. Despite the widespread use of IV iron in patients with chronic kidney disease, there remains a concern that exposing patients to IV iron over a period of time may increase the risk of cardiovascular and infectious

Onyekachi Ifudu (ed.), Renal Anemia: Conflicts and Controversies, 115–121.
© 2002 Kluwer Academic Publishers.

morbidity and mortality. Two retrospective analyses of large numbers of Medicare patients, one retrospective analysis of patients from a large dialysis provider and one large prospective trial recently brought this issue to the forefront. This paper reviews these analyses along with the results of an international taskforce of experts in various specialties including renal medicine, erythropoiesis, cytokine biology adaptive immunity, and outcomes research who provided a recent consensus on this issue.

Iron and infectious risk

Iron is an essential element for bacteria growth and iron deprivation in bacterial cultures has been associated with inhibition of bacterial growth. Injection of inorganic iron into rodent models of bacterial infection enhances the virulence (*in vivo*) of many bacteria [3]. *In vitro* studies have demonstrated that free iron suppresses polymorphonuclear leukocyte phagocytosis [3,4]. Experimental pyelonephritis in mice has been exacerbated by the administration of IV iron as shown by increased bacterial growth and increased severity of lesions in the kidney [5]. The overall evidence suggests that iron increases bacterial virulence and decreases host defense mechanisms. These observations in addition to others suggest that severe iron overload or excessive parenteral iron therapy may increase infection risk and severity.

Several prospective and retrospective clinical trials have also found an association between iron overload (as defined by ferritin levels greater than 500–1000 ng/ml) and increased incidence of infection [6]. Most of these studies were performed before routine parenteral iron use was advocated by clinical practice guidelines [7]. A more recent prospective study evaluated the epidemiologic pattern of bacteremia in 988 patients receiving hemodialysis [8]. This study looked for, but did not find an association with parenteral iron supplementation. Only 5% of patients in this study had ferritin levels greater than 1000 ng/ml and a much higher percentage were on rHuEPO therapy. Thus iron overload was not a risk factor for infection in this more recent cohort of patients.

However, two observational analyses by Collins and colleagues found an association between parenteral iron use and infections in a large cohort of US Medicare patients. The first study evaluated Medicare claims data in 33,120 prevalent hemodialysis patients in 1994 [9]. Patients were divided into two groups based on IV iron utilization (low group: 1–3 months of IV iron, high group: 4–6 months of IV iron) in the six month entry period. A Cox regression analysis was used adjusting for age, race, gender, 11 comorbid conditions, number of PRBC transfusions, vascular access procedures, hospital days, mean hematocrit level and prior ESRD duration. The results showed an 8% higher risk of all-cause death in the high frequency group and a 35% higher risk of infectious death. Following this analysis, new data showed that bacteremia in dialysis patients correlated with dialysis catheter use and prior hospitalizations for bacteremia. Collins and colleagues performed a second analysis using 1994 and 1995 prevalent hemodialysis patients and excluded patients with dialysis catheters and/or prior hospitalizations for bacteremia or sepsis [10]. In this analyses they evaluated the number of IV iron vials administered during the six month entry period. The groups were broken into 1–6, 7–11, 12–17 and >17 vials. Similar covariates to the first study were used in this analysis. Patients who received >17 vials of iron during the six-month period had higher all-cause infectious and cardiac mortality risk.

The conclusions were that large doses of iron over 3–6 months may be a concern for patient safety. These retrospective studies provided evidence that there was an association between larger numbers of iron vials administered over relatively short periods of time. The limitations of this study included the inability to evaluate the actual dose administered, although during this time period standard practice was to infuse mg of IV iron per administration.

However, Feldman and colleagues performed a similar analysis using a clinical data set from Frescenius Medical Corporation, which contained IV iron doses, to examine the relationship between iron administration over a six-month period in 1996 [11]. There were 28,287 patients alive in 1996 with complete comorbidity profiles (age, gender, bicarbonate, albumin, phosphorus, hemoglobin, urea reduction rate, length of ESRD and diabetes). Iron use was evaluated over a six-month period and was categorized as none, less than 1000 mg and greater than 1000 mg. Sixty-three percent of patients received iron sometime in the six-month period. Consistent with prior findings from an analysis they performed in 1993 with Dialysis Morbidity and Mortality Study data, there was no evidence for enhanced risk of death with administration of 1000 mg over 6 months. However, doses of greater than 1000 mg over six months were associated with an elevated risk of death.

Retrospective analyses, such as the studies presented above, showed associations with frequent use, higher doses or vials of IV iron and an increased risk of death. It is important to remember that they do not demonstrate causality. Although in all of these studies, adjustments were made for several comorbidities, the higher risk associated with larger IV iron doses or vials may be related to unidentified residual confounders, especially from unmeasured covariates in the follow-up period.

There has been one large prospective randomized trial, which has evaluated the effects of normal as compared to low hematocrit levels in 1233 hemodialysis patients with cardiac disease receiving rHuEPO [12]. After 29 months of evalation, the study was discontinued early because there were higher numbers of deaths and first nonfatal myocardial infarctions in patients in the normal hematocrit group (goal hematocrit 42%) as compared with the low hematocrit (goal hematocrit: 30%) group. The results of this study were completed unexpected and there does not appear to be a single explanation for the results. An evaluation of hematocrit values and rHuEPO doses within each group did not show an association of higher hematocrit levels or higher rHuEPO doses with greater mortality. This study did not directly evaluate the relationship between IV iron use and mortality as this was an interventional trial evaluating the effects of rHuEPO on achieving higher hematocrits. However, IV iron was administered to significantly more patients in the higher hematocrit group as compared to the lower hematocrit group. Among patients in the normal hematocrit group who were studied for at least six months, logistic-regression analysis yielded an odds ratio of mortality of 2.4 ($p < 0.001$) for patients receiving IV iron during the six months before death or censoring. Those patients who survived in this group received on average 152 mg of iron dextran per four week period as compared to 214 mg among those who died. Again, this study was not designed to evaluate the effects of IV iron administration on mortality, so these post-hoc observations have limited validity.

Recently, in response to these reports and the unconfirmed perception that certain doses or dosing patterns of IV iron may be dangerous in CKD patients, an international taskforce of experts in nephrology, cytokine biology, erythropoiesis, interventional trials and outcomes research was convened [13]. They used analyses of the peer-reviewed literature, unpublished experimental results and professional experience to develop consensus recommendations on the following topics:

• Review of key literature associated with iron-related complications

• Chain of logic behind the National Kidney Foundation's Dialysis Outcomes Quality Initiative (NKF-DOQI) anemia clinical practice guidelines on repletion and maintenance therapy with iron

- Role of iron as a provocateur for infectious complications and/or as an accelerant for cardiovascular disease

- Utility and limitations of currently available measures of iron status

- Population-based, cohort studies of iron-related complications

- Iron-related secondary outcomes in prospective, interventional trials

- Novel retrospective and intervention analyses to further expand knowledge in this area

A series of eight articles address the main points of these analyses [4,6,14–19]. It was the taskforce consensus that the NKF-DOQI clinical practice guidelines on iron management contain appropriate interventions and performances measures for the management of iron therapy in CKD patients with anemia. They urged that the dialysis care team routinely monitor hemoglobin, percent transferrin saturation (TSAT) and serum ferritin concentrations.

Parenteral iron remains the preferred therapy of repletion and maintenance therapy in these patients, but the therapy should be discontinued if the TSAT is above 50% and/or serum ferritin concentration is above 800 ng/ml. They emphasized the point that good clinical practice suggests that IV iron should be withheld in any patient with an active infection. There is not enough substantive information to without IV iron from other patient groups such as those with significant cardiovascular disease or prior history of infection. They noted that there were enough positive retrospective and prospective investigations of sufficient merit that suggested IV iron use may be deleterious in some CKD patients that additional studies need to be undertaken to provide further evidence.

There are several questions that still need to be addressed in the area of iron management in patients with CKD. 1) Is there a role for oxygen scavengers such as vitamin E or melatonin [20] to lower the potential increased risk of mortality associated with IV iron? 2) Is there a role for ascorbic acid [21,22] to enhance efficacy of rHuEPO while decreasing possible risks of IV iron therapy? 3) Are there specific doses or patterns of IV iron use that predispose patients to increased risks of morbidity or mortality?

Both rHuEPO and iron are necessary to sustain adequate erythropoiesis in patients with CKD. Since oral iron has shown little efficacy in the CKD population, IV iron therapy has become the mainstay of iron management in this population [2]. Clinicians should continue to follow the K/DOQI guidelines on management of anemia with rHuEPO and iron therapy to achieve target hematocrit levels of 33–36% [2]. Further studies which evaluate the risks and benefits of various IV iron dosages and dosing patterns as well as adjuvant therapy such as ascorbic acid, vitamin E and melatonin need to be undertaken.

REFERENCES

1. Eschbach JW, Adamson JW. Iron overload in renal failure patients: changes since the introduction of erythropoietin therapy. Kidney Int. 1999;69:S35–S43.
2. Anonymous. National Kidney Foundation. K/DOQI Clinical Practice Guidelines for Anemia of Chronic Kidney Disease, 2000. Am J Kidney Dis. 2001;37:S182–S238.
3. Patruta SI, Horl WH. Iron and infection. Kidney Int. 1999;69(supplement):S125–30.
4. Sunder-Plassmann G, Patruta SI, Horl WH. Pathobiology of the role of iron in infection. Am J Kidney Dis. 1999;34:S25–9.
5. Ang O, Gungor M, Aricioglu F, Inanc D, Sagduyu H, Uysal v, et al. The effect of parenteral iron administration on the development of Staphylococcus aureus-induced experimental pyelonephritis in rats. Int J Exp Pathol. 1990;71:507–11.
6. Hoen B. Iron and infection: clinical experience. Am J Kidney Dis. 1999;34:S30–4.
7. Anonymous. NKF-DOQI clinical practice guidelines for the treatment of anemia of chronic renal failure. National Kidney Foundation-Dialysis Outcomes Quality Initiative. Am J Kidney Dis. 1997;30:S192–S240.
8. Hoen B, Paul-Dauphin A, Hestin D, Kessler M. EPIBACDIAL: a multicenter prospective study of risk factors for baceremia in chronic hemodialysis patients. J Am Soc Nephrol. 1998;9:869–76.
9. Collins A, Ebben J, Ma J. Frequent IV iron dosing is associated with higher infectious deaths. J Am Soc Nephrol. 1997;8:190A (Abstract).
10. Collins A, Ebben J, Ma J, Xia A. I.V. iron dosing patterns and mortality. J Am Soc Nephrol. 1998;9:205A (Abstract).
11. Feldman HI, Santana J, Franklin E, Joffe M, Guo W, Faich G. Iron administration and survival in chronic hemodialysis patients. J Am Soc Nephrol. 2000;11:230A (Abstract).
12. Besarab A, Bolton WK, Browne JK, Egrie JC, Nissenson AR, Okamoto DM, et al. The effects of normal as compared with low hematocrit values in patients with cardiac disease who are receiving hemodialysis and epoetin. N Engl J Med. 1998; 339:584–90.
13. Owen WF, Jr. Optimizing the use of parenteral iron in end-stage renal disease patients: focus on issues of infection and cardiovascular disease. Introduction. Am J Kidney Dis. 1999;34:S1–S2.
14. Besarab A. Iron and cardiac disease in the end-stage renal disease setting. Am J Kidney Dis. 1999;34:S18–S24.
15. Fishbane S. Review of issues relating to iron and infection. Am J Kidney Dis. 1999;34:S47–S52.
16. Bistrian BR, Khaodhiar L. The systemic inflammatory response and its impact on iron nutriture in end-stage renal disease. Am J Kidney Dis. 1999;34:S35–9.

17. Cavill I. Iron status as measured by serum ferritin: the marker and its limitations. Am J Kidney Dis. 1999;34:S12–S17.
18. Macdougall IC, Chandler G, Elston O, Harchowal J. Beneficial effects of adopting an aggressive intravenous iron policy in a hemodialysis unit. Am J Kidney Dis. 1999;34:S40–6.
19. Owen WF, Szczech L, Johnson C, Frankenfield D. National perspective on iron therapy as a clinical performance measures for maintenance hemodialysis patients. Am J Kidney Dis. 1999;34:S5–S11.
20. Herrera J, Nava M, Romero F, Rodriguez-Iturbe B. Melatonin prevents oxidative stress resulting from iron and erythropoietin administration. Am J Kidney Dis. 2001;37:750–7.
21. Tarng DC, Wei YH, Huang TP, Kuo BI, Yang WC. Intravenous ascorbic acid as an adjuvant therapy for recombinant erythropoietin in hemodialysis patients with hyperferritinemia. Kidney Int. 1999;55:2477–86.
22. Tarng DC, Huang TP. A parallel, comparative study of intravenous iron versus intravenous ascorbic acid for erythropoietin-hyporesponsive anaemia in haemodialysis patients with iron overload. Nephrol Dial Transplantation. 1998;3:2867–72.

13. Anemia and erythropoietin therapy in kidney transplant recipients: where are the data?

Onyekachi Ifudu

INTRODUCTION

Prior to the availability of recombinant erythropoietin (EPO) [1], the mainstay of anemia therapy in end-stage renal disease (ESRD) were largely ineffective androgen injections and blood transfusions [2]. The latter carried significant risks of viral hepatitis infection, iron overload and sensitization to HLA antigens which often precludes being matched for a suitable cadaveric kidney transplant. In addition to correcting anemia, EPO therapy permits reduction or elimination of blood transfusion in ESRD patients thus a key beneficial effect of EPO treatment was less HLA sensitization with improved outcomes in kidney transplantation.

Despite these potential benefits, initially there were concerns that EPO may be immunomodulatory and may adversely affect renal allograft outcomes [3,4]. This review will examine the pathogenesis of anemia in kidney transplant recipients, and issues related to the use of EPO to correct anemia in this population.

Does pre-transplant EPO therapy jeorpardize renal allografts?

Following the wide spread use of EPO for anemia correction in ESRD patients receiving dialysis, there were concerns that EPO therapy may negatively impact outcomes in kidney transplant recipients. Based on animal and human studies showing that EPO increased immune activity, it was speculated that previous treatment with EPO may be associated with delayed graft function, and/or increased rate of graft rejection [3,4]. Also, because of increased viscosity that may accompany increased red cell mass there were concerns that EPO treatment may lead to graft loss due to blood clots [5].

Onyekachi Ifudu (ed.), Renal Anemia: Conflicts and Controversies, 123–128.
© 2002 *Kluwer Academic Publishers.*

However, several studies have shown that treatment with EPO had no negative impact on graft function or survival [5–10]. Paganini et al. [9], reported no difference in need for posttransplant dialysis support or severity of posttransplant acute renal failure between patients who had previously received EPO and those who did not. In a study of 120 consecutive renal transplant recipients, 58% of whom received prior EPO treatment, it was found that the incidence of acute rejection, time to first rejection and 1-year graft survival rate did not differ between those who received EPO and those who did not [8]. In fact, Linde et al. [10], showed that pretransplant EPO treatment aimed at reaching a normal hemoglobin reduces the postoperative requirement for blood transfusions and has no deleterious effects on kidney graft function.

Furthermore, anemia correction with EPO did not accelerate progression in chronic graft dysfucntion [6,7]. Thus, despite the initial concerns of an immunomodulatory effect of EPO available clinical evidence show that prior treatment with EPO does not increase incidence of delayed graft function, acute rejections or rate of progression of chronic allograft loss. Investigators have also found no association between primary renal graft thrombosis and pretransplant treatment with EPO [5].

Endogenous erythropoietin and post-transplant erythropoiesis

Endogenous erythropoietin is a glycoprotein hormone of primarily renal origin that promotes the proliferation and differentiation of erythrocyte precursors. In situ hybridization studies have shown that erythropoietin production in the hypoxic kidney occurs primarily in peritubular cells, most likely endothelial cells.

In transplant recipients, serum erythropoietin returns to normal as the hematocrit level increases to greater than 32% [11]. Thereafter, the hematocrit continues to increase to normal levels, while serum erythropoietin remains in the normal range [11]. Moderately increased blood levels of endogenous erythropoietin usually induce complete correction of anemia after successful kidney transplantation [11–13]. Evidence from new kidney transplant recipients suggest that slight increases in renal endogenous erythropoietin levels induce erythropoiesis to the same extent as do large doses of exogenous erythropoietin [11–13]. With good graft function, erythropoiesis is maintained by "normal" serum erythropoietin levels [11–13].

The key determinants of the serum level of endogenous erythropoietin among kidney transplant recipients is unclear. Erythropoietin level does not precisely correlate with amount of renal function. An early peak in serum erythropoietin level has been observed within two days of kidney transplantation in recipients with delayed graft function [14,15], suggesting that a nonuremic environment is not a prerequisite for production of erythropoietin [16]. However, this peak in erythropoietin level failed to induce an increase in hematocrit [15].

In fact, anemia failed to improve in some kidney transplant recipients despite a nine fold increase in endogenous erythropoietin level – hematocrit only began to rise with restoration of renal function [11,17]. Thus, restoration of renal excretory function, not ambient erythropoietin level appears to be the dominant factor that improves anemia in new kidney transplant recipients [15]. Indicating that extraction of uremic inhibitors plays a significant role in ameliorating anemia by enhancing the response of the bone marrow to modest levels of erythropoietin. Furthermore, previous treatment of dialysis patients with EPO does not blunt production of endogenous erythropoietin posttransplant or their ability to respond to EPO [9,18].

Is EPO safe in kidney transplant recipients?

Anemia is present in an unspecified though significant proportion of kidney transplant recipients, prompting the use of EPO [19]. Persistent anaemia (hematocrit $\leqslant 30\%$) in kidney transplant recipients may be associated with delayed graft function, acute or chronic allograft rejection, iron deficiency or blood loss [19–24] A rapid decrease in the body iron stores may accompany the brisk erythropoiesis that accompanies kidney transplantation [19,24], especially if such patients had inadequate iron stores while on maintenance dialysis. Furthermore, endogenous erythropoietin production may be diminished in some kidney transplant recipients despite normal allograft function [21]. For unknown reasons, anemia has persisted in some kidney transplant recipients with normal endogenous erythropoietin levels and normal allograft function [21].

EPO is effective in correcting anemia in kidney transplant recipients either in the immediate posttransplant period or among patients with failing renal allografts [20,22]. In a prospective randomized study to evaluate the efficacy of EPO during the first weeks after renal transplantation, Van Loo et al. [22], treated 14 patients with EPO subcutaneously (150 U/Kg/week) and compared them to a control group of 15 patients. In the group that received EPO, hematocrit increased from a mean of $22 \pm 4\%$ two weeks after transplantation to $30 \pm 4\%$ at week 4 and to $36 \pm 4\%$ at week 6 ($p < 0.001$ and $p < 0.0001$ respectively vs week 2). Corresponding values in the untreated group were $25 \pm 6\%$ at week 2, $28 \pm 6\%$ at week 4

(p = NS) and $32 \pm 6\%$ at week 6 ($p < 0.05$ vs week 2) (overall evolution EPO vs no EPO: $p = 0.038$ by ANOVA). The investigators concluded that EPO treatment effectively and safely corrects anemia during the first weeks after transplantation [22]. In a study of 40 patients with failing renal allografts, mean hemoglobin rose from 78.9 ± 10.4 to 102.6 ± 18.4 g/L after 24 weeks of treatment with EPO administered subcutaneously at a dose of 50 U/kg thrice weekly [20]. The amelioration of anemia was accompanied by significant improvements in global Sickness Impact Profile scores and in four of five dimensions of the Transplant Disease Questionnaire. The investigators reported no change in mean systolic or diastolic blood pressure but noted an increased need for antihypertensive drugs in eighteen study subjects [20].

The accompanying rise in hematocrit does not appear to either prolong the period of delayed graft function or accelerate loss of renal function among those kidney transplant recipients with chronic allograft dysfunction [20,22,25].

Predictors of response to EPO in kidney transplant recipients

The propensity of specific immunosuppressive agents to affect the action of EPO in kidney transplant recipients is unclear [7]. Either *in vitro* or animal studies utilizing single drug regimens are needed to clarify which of the commonly used immunosuppressive agents suppress marrow erythropoiesis or interfere with the actions of EPO.

The observed increase in endogenous erythropoietin in kidney transplant recipients treated with azathioprine has been attributed to a compensatory phenomenon to bone marrow suppression [26]. However, no difference was observed over time in neither the glomerular filtration rate nor the attained hematocrit in transplant patients randomized to receive azathioprine or cylcosporine [26]. Also, azathioprine may be associated with macrocytic anemia in some kidney transplant patients and anemia is more likely when azathioprine is used in combination with an angiotensin converting enzyme inhibitor [27].

There is an inverse correlation between EPO dose and creatinine clearance in kidney transplant recipients with chronic allograft dysfunction treated with EPO for anemia [20]. A sudden change in hematocrit in an EPO-treated transplant recipient may indicate declining graft function, blood loss, infection or iron deficiency [28]. Also, response to EPO is impaired during episodes of acute graft rejection, but is usually restored once rejection is successfully treated [28,29].

Does anemia affect long-term graft survival in kidney transplantation?

The prevalence of anemia in kidney transplant recipients is unknown. Though anemia may be present in many persons with normal graft function, it is clearly more prevalent among those with declining graft function [19,20]. In kidney transplant patients, neither the threshold hematocrit for initiation of EPO therapy nor the target hematocrit is established. Such paucity of data on anemia management and clinical use of EPO in kidney transplant recipients raises the question of whether current anemia management practices in the transplant population jeopardizes patient well-being ?

In addition to defining a threshold hematocrit that should prompt EPO therapy in kidney transplant recipients, key research questions that need to be addressed include; a) Does anemia correction positively impact outcome in kidney transplant recipients?, and b) Does renal anemia accelerate progression of chronic allograft loss in kidney transplant recipients?

REFERENCES

1. Eschbach JW, Abdulhadi MH, Browne JK, Delano BG, et al. Recombinant human erythropoietin in anemic patients with end-stage renal disease: results of a phase III multicenter clinical trial. Ann Intern Med. 1989;111:992–1000.
2. Koch KM, Patyna WD, Shaldon S, Werner E. Anemia of the regular hemodialysis patient and its treatment. Nephron. 1974;12:405–19.
3. Imiela J, Korczak-Kowalska G, Malecki R, Nowaczyk M, Stepien-Sopniewska B, Gorski A. Immunomodulatory action of human recombinant erythropoietin in man. Immunol Lett. 1993;35(3):271–5.
4. Singh AB, Singh M, Palekar S, Levy S, Nunn C, Mann RA. The effects of recombinant human erythropoietin on the cell mediated immune response of renal failure patients. J Med. 1992;23(5):289–302.
5. Bakir N, Sluiter WJ, Ploeg RJ, van Son WJ, Tegzess AM. Primary renal graft thrombosis. Nephrol Dial Transplantation. 1996;11(1):140–7.
6. Vanrenterghem Y, Vanwalleghem J. Benefits and concerns of treating pre-dialysis and renal transplant patients with recombinant human erythropoietin. Nephrol Dial Transplantation. 1998;13(supplement 2):13–5.
7. Lezaic V, Djukanovic L, Pavlovic-Kentera V. Recombinant human erythropoietin treatment of anemia in renal transplant patients. Renal Failure. 1995;17(6): 705–14.
8. Vasquez EM, Pollak R. Effect of pretransplant erythropoietin therapy on renal allograft outcome. Transplantation. 1996;15;62(7):1026–8.
9. Paganini EP, Braun WE, Latham D, Abdulhadi MH. Renal transplantation: results in hemodialysis patients previously treated with recombinant human erythropoietin. ASAIO Trans. 1989;35(3):535–8.
10. Linde T, Ekberg H, Forslund T, Furuland H, Holdaas H, Nyberg G, Tyden G, Wahlberg J, Danielson BG. The use of pretransplant erythropoietin to normalize

hemoglobin levels has no deleterious effects on renal transplantation outcome. Transplantation. 2001;71(1):79–82.

11. Wolff M, Jelkmann W. Erythropoiesis and erythropoietin levels in renal transplant recipients. Klin Wochenschr. 1991;69:53–8.

12. Sun CH, Ward HJ, Paul WL, et al. Serum erythropoietin levels after renal transplantation. N Engl J Med. 1989;321:151–7.

13. Lee DB. Interrelationship between erythropoietin and erythropoiesis: insights from renal transplantation. Am J Kidney Dis. 1991;18:54–6.

14. Beshara S, Birgegard G, Goch J, Wahlberg J, Wikstrom B, Danielson BG. Assessment of erythropoiesis following renal transplantation. Eur J Haematol. 1997;58(3):167–73.

15. Brown JH, Lappin TR, Elder GE, Taylor TN, Bridges JM, McGeown MG. The initiation of erythropoiesis following renal transplantation. Nephrol Dial Transplantation. 1989;4(12):1076–9.

16. Eckhardt KU, Frei U, Kliem V, Bauer C, Koch KM, Kurtz A. Role of excretory graft function for erythropoietin formation after renal transplantation. Eur J Clin Invest. 1990;20(5):563–72.

17. Besarab A, Caro J, Jarrell BE, Francos G, Erslev AJ. Dynamics of erythropoiesis following renal transplantation. Kidney Int. 1987;32(4):526–36.

18. Fernandez Lucas M, Marcen R, Villafruela J, Teruel JL, Tato A, Rivera M, Ortuno J. Effect of rHuEpo therapy in dialysis patients on endogenous erythropoietin synthesis after renal transplantation. Nephron. 1996;73(1):54–7.

19. Miles AM, Markell MS, Daskalakis P, et al. Anemia following renal transplantation: erythropoietin response and iron deficiency. Clin Transplant. 1997;11:313–5.

20. Muirhead N, Cattran DC, Zaltzman J, et al. Safety and efficacy of recombinant human erythropoietin in correcting the anaemia of patients with chronic renal allograft dysfunction. J Am Soc Nephrol. 1994;5:1216–22.

21. Nampoory MR, Johny KV, al-Hilali N, et al. Erythropoietin deficiency and relative resistance cause anaemia in post-renal transplant recipients with normal renal function. Nephrol Dial Transplantation. 1996;11:177–81.

22. Van Loo A, Vanholder R, Bernaert P, et al. Recombinant human erythropoietin corrects anaemia during the first weeks after renal transplantation: a randomized prospective study. Nephrol Dial Transplantation. 1996;11:1815–21.

23. Almond MK, Tailor D, Marsh FP, et al. Increased erythropoietin requirements in patients with failed renal transplants returning to a dialysis programme. Nephrol Dial Transplantation. 1994;9:270–3.

24. Tornero F, Prats D, Alvarez-Sala JL, Coronel F, Sanchez A, Barrientos A. Iron deficiency anemia after successful renal transplantation. J Urol. 1993;149(6):1398–400.

25. Traindl O, Barnas U, Franz M, Falger S, Klauser R, Kovarik J, Graf H. Recombinant human erythropoietin in renal transplant recipients with renal anemia. Clin Transplant. 1994;8(1):45–8.

26. Jensen JD, Hansen HE, Pedersen EB.Increased serum erythropoietin level during azathioprine treatment in renal transplant recipients. Nephron. 1994;67(3):297–301.

27. Gossmann J, Kachel HG, Schoeppe W, Scheuermann EH. Anemia in renal transplant recipients caused by concomitant therapy with azathioprine and angiotensin-converting enzyme inhibitors. Transplantation. 1993;56(3):585–9.

28. Aufricht C, Marik JL, Ettenger RB. Subcutaneous recombinant human erythropoietin in chronic renal allograft dysfunction. Pediatr Nephrol. 1998;12(1):10–3.

29. Page B, Zingraff J. Resistance to rHuEpo and kidney graft rejection. Nephrol Dial Transplantation. 1994;9(11):1696.

14. Intravenous iron treatment: a comparison of available drugs

Steven Fishbane

INTRODUCTION

Iron supplementation is an important component of anemia treatment for patients on hemodialysis. Iron deficiency develops in these patients for three primary reasons. First, chronic blood loss related to dialysis apparatus blood retention, accidental and surgical blood loss and blood testing [1–3]. Second, the use of phosphate binders interferes with dietary iron absorption [3]. Third, epoetin alfa treatment stimulates rapid production of red blood cells, creating a deficiency of immediately available circulating iron [4–5]. The net result is that iron deficiency is common in hemodialysis patients, and is an important factor that may hinder the achievement of target hemoglobin levels [6].

Oral iron treatment had been a mainstay of anemia therapy for patients on dialysis for the first 5 years that epoetin alfa therapy was available. Starting in 1995, a series of studies demonstrated that intravenous iron had demonstrably greater efficacy than oral iron [7–9]. Moreover, at least 3 published studies in hemodialysis patients have examined oral iron treatment in relation to a placebo or no iron control group [10–12]. None of these studies found any efficacy of oral iron treatment in this patient population. In addition, oral iron treatment leads to frequent gastrointestinal complaints [13]. As a result, published anemia practice guidelines in the United States and Europe have downplayed the use of oral iron [14,15].

Intravenous iron treatment has emerged as the favored method for maintaining and replacing iron in hemodialysis patients. In the US there are currently three types of intravenous iron currently available, iron dextran, sodium ferric gluconate complex and iron sucrose. The purpose of this article is to critically compare these agents. I will discuss what is

Onyekachi Ifudu (ed.), Renal Anemia: Conflicts and Controversies, 129–138.
© *2002 Kluwer Academic Publishers.*

known of the efficacy and safety of each, and use this information to synthesize a rational approach to the use of the drugs.

Iron dextran

Iron dextran has been used in the US for many years for the treatment of iron deficiency. The steric structure is analogous to that of ferritin [3]. The body uses ferritin to safely contain iron and hold it tightly in storage until needed. To do so, ferritin compacts iron into a dense central core in the form of iron oxyhydroxide [16]. This is the same core structure used in iron dextran. Ferritin surrounds the iron core with protein, apoferritin, and iron dextran surrounds the core with glucose polymers termed dextran chains. Iron dextran is believed to tightly bind its central iron core [17].

Dextran chains were first used in clinical medicine as volume expanders. They were effective for the purpose, but occasional episodes of anaphylaxis were reported [18]. Indeed, the major problem with the use of iron dextran has been related to allergy and anaphylaxis. Serious allergic reactions have been found to occur in 0.6% to 0.7% of hemodialysis patients treated with the drug [19–20]. For individual patients the risk is thus quite low, but on a population basis the effect is quite significant. It is estimated that approximately 60% of hemodialysis patients are treated with intravenous iron in a year. For a base of 200,000 patients, if 120,000 were treated with iron dextran then approximately 700 patients would have reactions severe enough to require hospitalization. In fact, over the past ten years there have been 31 reported deaths due to iron dextran [21].

The mechanism of these reactions is not fully known. The clinical syndrome of anaphylaxis occurs because of an explosive release of mediators from mast cells and basophils. This is believed to occur with iron dextran related anaphylaxis, but the underlying stimulus is unclear. Neither IgE nor immune complexes seem to play an important role. It may be that there is a direct stimulation of mast cell release, similar to what is found with opiate or contrast media induced anaphylaxis [22].

The efficacy of intravenous iron dextran has been evaluated in several published studies. One use of the drug is for replacement of iron stores for absolute iron deficiency, when the serum ferritin is less than 100 ng/ml. In this setting we found the drug to be consistently effective. Mean hematocrit levels increased from $29.1 \pm 0.9\%$ at baseline to $33.6 \pm 1.8\%$ ($p < 0.05$) and the mean erythropoietin dose decreased from 94.1 ± 5.3 U/kg body weight to 82.6 ± 4.4 U ($p < 0.05$) [23]. Studies of iron dextran for chronic maintenance of iron stores have similarly demonstrated consistent efficacy [7–9]. Thus, on balance iron dextran is a drug with excellent efficacy but with an important risk of severe allergic reactions.

Sodium ferric gluconate complex

This drug has been used in Europe for several decades, primarily in Italy and Germany. It was approved by the US Food and Drug Administration in February of 1999, and has been used widely in the US since then. The iron is in the form of iron saccharate, with a gluconate moiety that bridges the iron centers. The molecular weight appears to be 350,000 daltons which is significantly larger than iron dextran. The drug is certainly large enough so that it is not dialyzable and may be administered at any time during the hemodialysis treatment.

Several published studies have evaluated the efficacy of intravenous sodium ferric gluconate in hemodialysis patients. Allegra et al. treated patients with 31.25 mg at each hemodialysis treatment for 6 months. They found improved hemoglobin concentrations despite the fact that patients did not receive epoetin treatment [24]. Navarro et al. found the administration of sodium ferric gluconate to be safe and efficient in maintaining adequate body iron stores [25]. Taylor et al. studied patients during stable epoetin therapy. Patients were treated with 62.5 mg of ferric gluconate once or twice weekly, or once every two weeks. The results demonstrated a significant improvement in hemoglobin concentration and reduction in epoetin dose requirements.

In addition, many of the study patients had a normal serum ferritin concentration at baseline, and even among these patients there was a significant improvement in epoetin response, with a mean dose reduction of 33% while the mean serum hemoglobin increased by 1.3 g/dl [26]. Similar positive findings were reported by Braun et al. [27], Cortes et al. [28], Pascual et al. [29], Nissenson et al. [30] and Fudin et al. [11].

Taken together, the existing literature up to 2001 indicated excellent efficacy of sodium ferric gluconate. It is in safety that the drug appears to be greatly superior to iron dextran. In an interesting epidemiological study in 1999, the safety of iron dextran and ferric gluconate were compared via a review of spontaneous adverse reaction reporting to the World Health Organization, pharmaceutical manufacturers, and the German Health Bureau. The number of exposures to ferric gluconate was estimated to be 2.5 million per year from 1976 to 1996, a rate similar to iron dextran use in the US. During this time period not a single death was reported involving treatment with ferric gluconate. In comparison, 31 deaths were reported with the use of iron dextran during a shorter ten year period [21].

This provided stark evidence to support the long-held anecdotal contention that this drug is significantly safer than iron dextran.

A large multicenter study was recently concluded, with partial results reported at the American Society of Nephrology meeting in October, 2000. Sixty-nine centers enrolled a total of 2534 patients who received double blind administration of sodium ferric gluconate complex and placebo. The drug was administered without a test dose and by intravenous push. The preliminary report of the first 1122 patients randomized indicated no significant difference in the rate of adverse reactions between sodium ferric gluconate and placebo. The drug was found to be quite safe in patients previously allergic to iron dextran (abstract, Eschbach et al., American Society of Nephrology, 2000). In the entire study there was only one life threatening reaction with sodium ferric gluconate among 2534 patients treated. This rate was not statistically different than that of placebo. When compared to iron dextran historical controls, the reduction in risk of a severe reaction was approximately 93% with sodium ferric gluconate. Moreover, the one life threatening reaction with sodium ferric gluconate in this study was over in 20 minutes, and the patient finished dialysis and went home afterwards (personal communication, S. Fishbane). This is in stark contrast to the catastrophic reactions seen with iron dextran.

Sodium ferric gluconate complex is, therefore, a major step forward in drug safety compared with iron dextran. A test dose is not needed prior to treatment, and slow intravenous push administration is safe and effective. Little is known however with respect to the maximum dose that can be administered at one time. However, three recent reports indicates that 250 mg by intravenous infuasion is safe and effective (abstract, Folkert et al., American Society of Nephrology, 2001, abstract, Wynn R, European Dialysis and Transplantation Association, 2001, abstract, Javier AM, European Dialysis and Transplantation Association, 2001).

One safety issue that was previously raised with sodium ferric gluconate complex regarded rapid release of iron. Zanen et al. found that after intravenous administration, serum iron concentration rose rapidly leading to oversaturation of transferrin [31]. Under these conditions toxic free iron could exist in the circulation. These results, however, were recently found to be highly flawed [32].

The problem relates to the method used for measuring serum iron concentration. The initial step in measuring serum iron is to add an agent to the serum sample to remove iron from transferrin. Zanen's technique for doing this was to acidify serum with ascorbic acid in guanidine [31]. In

Seligman and Schleicher's analysis, this method was found to release iron not only from transferrin, but also from the drug ferric gluconate [32]. Therefore, what Zanen reported as serum iron actually represented an important quantity of iron contained in the drug. Indeed, subsequent pharmacokinetic studies indicate that iron oversaturation does not occur with sodium ferric gluconate (personal communication, J. Strobos MD).

Iron sucrose

This agent contains iron as a polynuclear iron-sucrose complex [24]. The drug has been used extensively in Europe for decades, and received FDA approval in the US in November, 2000. While this drug has not been evaluated by a large randomized-blinded study as sodium ferric gluconate has, I believe that it probably shares many of that drug's favorable safety attributes. It should be noted that the terminology used to describe this drug in the literature is inconsistent and confusing. Some studies refer to iron saccharate compounds, others to iron sucrose, at is not always clear whether the drugs are the same.

Recently, Charytan et al. published a report of the pivotal North American trial. Seventy-seven hemodialysis patients were treated with ten consecutive doses of 100 mg of intravenous iron sucrose administered by 5 minute intravenous push. Serum hemoglobin was targeted at 11.0 g/dl, and 78% of patients reached that level. A statistically significant increase in serum hemoglobin level was achieved within 3 weeks of initiating therapy. No serious drug reactions or anaphylaxis were noted [33]. In a separate report from this trial, Van Wyck et al. noted that the drug was well tolerated in patients with previous iron dextran allergy. None of 23 such patients experienced allergy or anaphylaxis on treatment with iron sucrose [34].

Sunder-Plassmann and Horl studied the drug in 64 hemodialysis patients over a 22-month period. The dose used was 10–20 mg each dialysis session, with a brisk and sustained clinical response [9]. Similarly, Silverberg et al. demonstrated significant improvement in serum hemoglobin in both hemodialysis and peritoneal dialysis patients treated with intravenous iron sucrose [35]. In contrast, Stoves et al. recently studied the drug in comparison to oral iron among patients with progressive renal insufficiency. No benefit was demonstrated with the intravenous iron sucrose when given as 300 mg per month, when compared to oral ferrous sulfate administered as 600 mg per day [36]. Drug safety was evaluated in a study reported by Hoigne et al. in 1998, based on a group of 400 obstetric patients treated with iron sucrose. There were 7 generalized reactions, 4 with flushing and 3 with rash. In the same report, a retrospective study of hemodialysis patients was conducted by survey of dialysis medical directors. No life threatening reactions were reported from an estimated exposure of 8100 patient-years with administrations of a 100 mg dose. There were 5–7 episodes of hypotension, and 10 patients experienced flushing [37]. This study seems to support the anecdotal view of the excellent safety of this drug, consistent with most published studies. However, because most clinical trials with this drug have been of small size, further research on iron sucrose should focus on drug safety.

One concern with iron sucrose has been for the risk of the drug inducing osteomalacia [38–40]. Sato and Shiraki published an extensive review on this subject [38]. They hypothesize that saccharated iron impairs proximal renal tubular function, leading to renal phosphate wasting and hypophosphatemia. Osteomalacia observed in patients treated with iron sucrose appears due to the hypophosphatemia [38]. This is unlikely to be a problem for patients on dialysis given their greatly diminished glomerular filtration and tendency towards phosphate accumulation rather than depletion. It is unclear, because of inconsistent terminology in the literature, whether iron sucrose and saccharated iron are identical.

Another safety concern with iron sucrose relates to a potential risk for inducing infection. Parkkinen et al. found that injection of the drug led to the presence of catalytically active iron in the circulation. This was detected as bleomycin detectable iron after injection of 100 mg of iron sucrose in 7 of 12 patients studied. Moreover, patients' serum lost the ability to inhibit the growth of *Staphylococcus epidermidis*, but regained the ability after iron-free transferrin was added to the serum.

These findings suggest that iron sucrose, perhaps due to its small size, may release free iron too readily, and may predispose to infection [41]. This is supported by the recent work of Damiani et al., who found higher infection rates in patients treated with iron sucrose. These authors suggested that "quick" iron release for iron sucrose might be the problem (abstract, Damiani et al., European Dialysis and transplantation Association, 2001). The long-term positive safety record of iron sucrose would seem to conflict with these study findings. Clearly, given the importance of infection in dialysis patients, further research is necessary.

As to a maximum dose of iron sucrose that can be given at one time, there is little data to help in this regard. The FDA approved product label states that 100 mg is the maximum single dose. One recent report by Vychytil and Haag-Weber examined iron sucrose use in peritoneal dialysis patients. They found that 0.9% of patients receiving 100 mg, and 5.9%

Table 1.

Drug	Brand name(s)	Anaphylactic risk	Bolded label warnings	Test dose needed	Slow IV push	Maximum single dose
Sodium ferric gluconate complex	Ferrlecit®	Low	No	No	Yes	250 mg
Iron sucrose	Venofer®	Low	Yes	No	Yes	250 mg
Iron dextran	InFed® Dexferrum®	Moderate	Black Box	Yes	Yes	1000 mg

receiving 200 mg over ten minutes experienced reactions such as hypotension and back pain [42]. The authors concluded that a slower rate of infusion might be helpful. Similarly, Sunder-Plassmann and Horl recently recommended a maximum dose for iron sucrose of 100–200 mg [43]. My opinion is that like sodium ferric gluconate, intravenous iron sucrose should not be administered in doses greater than 250 mg at one time.

CONCLUSIONS (Table 1)

Sodium ferric gluconate complex and iron sucrose are considerably safer for use in hemodialysis patients than iron dextran. These drugs should mostly replace the use of iron dextran. The one setting in which iron dextran is still preferred is when large single doses are needed (> 250 mg). It is unclear that either sodium ferric gluconate or iron sucrose are well tolerated when given in these higher doses.

Additional research is needed to fully define clinical differences between sodium ferric gluconate and iron sucrose. The large randomized placebo-controlled safety trial for sodium ferric gluconate discussed above serves as an excellent model for such research. Other important areas for research include: 1) determining the maximum single doses that can be safely tolerated with sodium ferric gluconate and iron sucrose, 2) better defining issues related to iron release and infection with iron sucrose.

REFERENCES

1.   Bone JM. Blood loss and iron requirements in patients on haemodialysis. Scott Med J. 1972;17(8):264–5.
2.   Akmal M, Sawelson S, Karubian F, Gadallah M. The prevalence and significance of occult blood loss in patients with predialysis advanced chronic renal failure (CRF), or receiving dialytic therapy. Clin Nephrol. 1994;42(3):198–202.
3.   Fishbane S, Maesaka JK. Iron management in end-stage renal disease. Am J Kidney Dis. 1997;29(3):319–33.
4.   Brugnara C, Colella GM, Cremins J, Langley RC Jr, Schneider TJ, Rutherford CJ, Goldberg MA. Effects of subcutaneous recombinant human erythropoietin in normal subjects: development of decreased reticulocyte hemoglobin content and iron-deficient erythropoiesis. J Lab Clin Med. 1994;123(5):660–7.
5.   Rutherford CJ, Schneider TJ, Dempsey H, Kirn DH, Brugnara C, Goldberg MA. Efficacy of different dosing regimens for recombinant human erythropoietin in a simulated perisurgical setting: the importance of iron availability in optimizing response. Am J Med. 1994;96(2):139–45.
6.   Richardson D, Bartlett C, Will EJ. Optimizing erythropoietin therapy in hemodialysis patients. Am J Kidney Dis. 2001;38(1):109–17.

7. Fishbane S, Frei GL, Maesaka J. Reduction in recombinant human erythropoietin doses by the use of chronic intravenous iron supplementation. Am J Kidney Dis. 1995;26(1):41–6.

8. Sepandj F, Jindal K, West M, Hirsch D. Economic appraisal of maintenance parenteral iron administration in treatment of anaemia in chronic haemodialysis patients. Nephrol Dial Transplantation. 1996;11(2):319–22.

9. Sunder-Plassmann G, Horl WH. Importance of iron supply for erythropoietin therapy. Nephrol Dial Transplantation. 1995;10(11):2070–6.

10. Markowitz GS, Kahn GA, Feingold RE, Coco M, Lynn RI. An evaluation of the effectiveness of oral iron therapy in hemodialysis patients receiving recombinant human erythropoietin. Clin Nephrol. 1997;48(1):34–40.

11. Fudin R, Jaichenko J, Shostak A, Bennett M, Gotloib L. Correction of uremic iron deficiency anemia in hemodialyzed patients: a prospective study. Nephron. 1998; 79(3):299–305.

12. Macdougall IC, Tucker B, Thompson J, Tomson CR, Baker LR, Raine AE. A randomized controlled study of iron supplementation in patients treated with erythropoietin. Kidney Int. 1996;50(5):1694–9.

13. Macdougall IC. Strategies for iron supplementation: oral versus intravenous. Kidney Int. 1999;69:S61–6.

14. NKF-DOQI clinical practice guidelines for the treatment of anemia of chronic renal failure. National Kidney Foundation-Dialysis Outcomes Quality Initiative. Am J Kidney Dis. 1997;30(4 supplement 3):S192–240.

15. Cameron JS. European best practice guidelines for the management of anaemia in patients with chronic renal failure. Nephrol Dial Transplantation. 1999;14 (supplement 2):61–5.

16. Cowley JM, Janney DE, Gerkin RC, Buseck PR. The structure of ferritin cores determined by electron nanodiffraction. J Struct Biol. 2000;131(3):210–6.

17. Geisser P, Baer M, Schaub E. Structure/histotoxicity relationship of parenteral iron preparations. Arzneimittelforschung. 1992;42(12):1439–52.

18. Bailey G, Strub RL, Klein RC, Salvaggio J. Dextran-induced anaphylaxis. JAMA. 1967;200(10):889–91.

19. Fishbane S, Ungureanu VD, Maesaka JK, Kaupke CJ, Lim V, Wish J. The safety of intravenous iron dextran in hemodialysis patients. Am J Kidney Dis. 1996;28 (4):529–34.

20. Hamstra RD, Block MH, Schocket AL. Intravenous iron dextran in clinical medicine. JAMA. 1980;243(17):1726–31.

21. Faich G, Strobos G. Sodium ferric gluconate complex in sucrose: safer intravenous iron therapy than iron dextrans. Am J Kidney Dis. 1999;33(3):464–70.

22. Novey HS, Pahl M, Haydik I, Vaziri ND. Immunologic studies of anaphylaxis to iron dextran in patients on renal dialysis. Ann Allergy. 1994;72(3):224–8.

23. Fishbane S, Lynn RI. The efficacy of iron dextran for the treatment of iron deficiency in hemodialysis patients. Clin Nephrol. 1995;44(4):238–40.

24. Bailie GR, Johnson CA, Mason NA. Parenteral iron use in the management of anemia in end-stage renal disease patients. Am J Kidney Dis. 2000;35(1):1–12.

25. Navarro JF, Teruel JL, Liano F, Marcen R, Ortuno J. Effectiveness of intravenous administration of Fe-gluconate-Na complex to maintain adequate body iron stores in hemodialysis patients. Am J Nephrol. 1996;16:268–72.

26. Taylor JE, Peat N, Porter C, Morgan AG. Regular low-dose intravenous iron therapy improves response to erythropoietin in haemodialysis patients. Nephrol Dial Transplantation. 1996;11(6):1079–83.

27. Braun J, Lindner K, Schreiber M, Heidler RA, Hörl WH. Percentage of hypochromic red blood cells as predictor of erythropoietic and iron response after i.v. iron

supplementation in maintenance haemodialysis patients. Nephrol Dial Transplantation. 1997;12:1173–81.

28. Cortes MJC, Perales MCS, Utiel FJB, Serrano P, Del Barrio PP, Liebana A, Hinojosa JB, Marcos SG, Banasco VP. Effect of intravenous Na-Fe-gluconate in hemodialysis patients treating with rHuEPO. Nefrologia. 1997;17:424–9.

29. Pascual J, Teruel JL, Liano F, Sureda A, Ortuno J. Intravenous Fe-gluconate-Na for iron-deficient patients on hemodialysis. Nephron. 1992;60:121 (letter).

30. Nissenson AR, Lindsay RM, Swan S, Seligman P, Strobos J. Sodium ferric gluconate complex in sucrose is safe and effective in hemodialysis patients. N Am Clin Trial. Am J Kidney Dis. 1999;33:471–82.

31. Zanen AL, Adriaansen HJ, van Bommel EF, Posthuma R, Th de Jong GM. 'Oversaturation' of transferrin after intravenous ferric gluconate (Ferrlicet(R)) in haemodialysis patients. Nephrol Dial Transplantation. 1996;11:820–4.

32. Seligman PA, Schleicher RB. Comparison of methods used to measure serum iron in the presence of iron gluconate or iron dextran. Clin Chem. 1999;45(6 Pt 1):898–901.

33. Charytan C, Levin N, Al-Saloum M, Hafeez T, Gagnon S, Van Wyck DB. Efficacy and safety of iron sucrose for iron deficiency in patients with dialysis-associated anemia: North American clinical trial. Am J Kidney Dis. 2001;37(2):300–7.

34. Van Wyck DB, Cavallo G, Spinowitz BS, Adhikarla R, Gagnon S, Charytan C, Levin N. Safety and efficacy of iron sucrose in patients sensitive to iron dextran: North American clinical trial. Am J Kidney Dis. 2000;36(1):88–97.

35. Silverberg DS, Blum M, Peer G, Kaplan E, Iaina A. Intravenous ferric saccharate as an iron supplement in dialysis patients. Nephron. 1996;72(3):413–7.

36. Stoves J, Inglis H, Newstead CG. A randomized study of oral vs intravenous iron supplementation in patients with progressive renal insufficiency treated with erythropoietin. Nephrol Dial Transplantation. 2001;16(5):967–74.

37. Hoigne R, Breymann C, Kunzi UP, Brunner F. Parenteral iron therapy: problems and possible solutions. Schweiz Med Wochenschr. 1998;128(14):528–35.

38. Sato K, Shiraki M. Saccharated ferric oxide-induced osteomalacia in Japan: iron-induced osteopathy due to nephropathy. Endocr J. 1998;45(4):431–9.

39. Suzuki A, Ohoike H, Matsuoka Y, Irimajiri S. Iatrogenic osteomalacia caused by intravenous administration of saccharated ferric oxide. Am J Hematol. 1993;43(1):75–6.

40. Okada M, Imamura K, Iida M, Fuchigami T, Omae T. Hypophosphatemia induced by intravenous administration of Saccharated iron oxide. Klin Wochenschr. 1983;61(2):99–102.

41. Parkkinen J, von Bonsdorff L, Peltonen S, Gronhagen-Riska C, Rosenlof K. Catalytically active iron and bacterial growth in serum of haemodialysis patients after i.v. iron-saccharate administration. Nephrol Dial Transplantation. 2000;15(11):1827–34.

42. Vychytil A, Haag-Weber M. Iron status and iron supplementation in peritoneal dialysis patients. Kidney Int. 1999;69:S71–8.

43. Sunder-Plassmann G, Horl WH. Comparative look at intravenous iron agents: Pharmacology, efficacy, sand safety of iron dextran, iron saccharate and ferric gluconate. Semin Dial. 1999;12(4):243–8.

Epilogue

Eli A. Friedman

Irreversible kidney failure has been transformed from a hopeless disorder in which marginal life might be tenuously extended for weeks to months by protein restriction, to the present when the major concern focuses on life quality months to years after initiation of ESRD therapy. Appreciating the extraordinary impact of treatment with erythropoietin in functionally anephric peritoneal dialysis and hemodialysis patients, Ifudu convened diverse professionals with shared interest in the uremic patient and concentrated their attention on the remarkable positive change in rehabilitation potential imparted by recombinant erythropoietin.

Addressing key issues raised by the now universal inclusion of erythropoietin in ESRD regimens as well as its burgeoning deployment during earlier stages of renal impairment, conference participants reached only one overriding conclusion: Raising erythrocyte mass with recombinant erythropoietin treatment is desirable, safe, and indicated for every patient with azotemia-related anemia irrespective of the cause of renal insufficiency. Earlier fears that a normal hematocrit threatened cerebrovascular accidents, unmanageable hypertension, and accelerated loss of hemodialysis vascular access have not been substantiated. Unless indications of cardiovascular or cerebrovascular instability are evident and worrisome, striving for a normal hematocrit makes sense as well as a happier patient.

At variance with the positive consensus over the value of erythropoietin as an all purpose life booster for kidney patients, however, were strong disagreements over other aspects of anemia management. The value of oral iron to sustain iron stores during long-term erythropoietin treatment was characterized in assessments ranging from "worthless" to "routinely used" in the majority of dialysis patients in some programs. The extent to which intravenous iron should be first line therapy was strongly debated without conclusion other than that well expressed by St. Peter: "Well-

Onyekachi Ifudu (ed.), Renal Anemia: Conflicts and Controversies, 139–140.
© *2002 Kluwer Academic Publishers.*

designed studies need to be conducted which evaluate IV iron dosage and dosing patterns." Fishbane thought the controversy resolved concluding: "Intravenous iron treatment has emerged as the favored method for maintaining and replacing iron in hemodialysis patients."

While erythropoietin was shown by Brown et al. to enhance survival of erythrocytes, and blunt development of cardiovascular disease in kidney failure, as reported by Levin, the suggestion by Friedman that treatment with erythropoietin retards deterioration of renal function in progressive renal disorders must be regarded as speculative though attractive. Whether route, dosing frequency, and amount of erythropoietin injected is determined by governmental regulation as suggested by reimbursement regulations as posited by Charytan or is an individual decision made by each physician as advised by Besarab must be characterized as a still open question. Illustrating the continuing dynamic evolution of treatment protocols for erythropoietin is the description by Lindberg of the testing and introduction of darbepoetin alfa, a novel, long-acting erythropoietin that can be given subcutaneously. Broad scale clinical trials of darbepoetin alfa found that the addition of two sialic acid chains indeed augments the hormone's potency while retaining its remarkable safety. Should this early experience be confirmed, darbepoetin alfa may rapidly become the erythropoietin of choice.

Individuals entrapped by a life dependent on thrice weekly machine cleansing of nitrogenous wastes (maintenance hemodialysis), have prevailed as their doctors learned how to replace missing vitamin D and erythropoietin thereby reducing the risk of formerly inevitable bone and heart complications. Refinements in the erythropoietin molecule combined with enhanced understanding of how to optimize its use have reaped tangible benefits for dialysis patients that will soon be extended to those with retained though deteriorating renal function. It will be as intriguing to compare reports of anemia treatment two years hence with consensus thinking in 2001 discerning contrasts as great as that of the speed and capability of a Pentium 4 with that of the discarded Pentium 3.

Index